Probiotics

Become Leaky Gut Free With the Use of Probiotics

(Everything You Need to Know on Delectable Recipes That Also Heal Gut to Make Healthy Living)

Johnny Haywood

Published By **Chris David**

Johnny Haywood

Probiotics: Become Leaky Gut Free With the Use of Probiotics (Everything You Need to Know on Delectable Recipes That Also Heal Gut to Make Healthy Living)

ISBN   978-1-998038-56-5

Legal & Disclaimer

Table Of Contents

Chapter 1: What 'EXACTLY' are Probiotics

"Probiotic" comes from the mixture of two Latin words that are 'pro', which refers to "for" and "biotic," an adjective which is derived from the word "bios," that means "life". So 'probiotic' literally stands for "for life". Probiotics are living microorganisms (yeasts or bacteria) with a wide range of advantages to health if consumed in the right quantities and regularly. Simply put, they are good bacteria.

For a deeper knowledge of what the term "probiotics" means they are, it is important to realize the high quantity of bacteria within the human body of each being. Indeed, each of us typically has ten to twenty times the amount of organisms in our bodies. The bacteria we have in our bodies exceed the number of cells that make up our bodies. The body is home to around 400 kinds of microorganisms we're in contact with, and approximately 15% are extremely important to maintaining our overall health. [1] Different types of probiotics offer certain advantages for health. The human body is believed to contain the equivalent of a number of bacteria to all humans that ever existed on this globe.

The healthy balance of healthy and harmful bacteria accomplishes various things to our body. They first form an abdominal barrier so that the beneficial nutrients are absorbed, and then retained to be used by the body. They also block harmful chemicals out of our bodies. The presence of probiotics aids in optimizing the functioning of our intestinal tract by establishing an equilibrium in the amount of beneficial microorganisms in our intestinal walls, thus promoting the health of our body.

Why Do We Need Probiotics

Modern diets are poor in nutrition and are stuffed with carbohydrates, hydrogenated fats as well as salt, refined carbohydrates as well as chemical preservatives, and other harmful components. These are fillers that technically do not provide any benefit to the body.

Probiotics may be present in our bodies, they require to be maintained regularly, in order to prevent their depletion and provide less benefits. The importance of these microbes is not to be undervalued. They fight off negative bacteria and combat disease and increase the immune system. In other words they're the first protection against any undesirable invaders into our bodies.

Probiotics are also helpful in many aspects of digestion. They help to break down food and efficiently extracting valuable nutrients. Researchers and medical professionals have been increasingly stating that we should take probiotics in just like we do vitamins. From minor health issues such as the common cold, to more serious illnesses like cancer, the consumption of probiotics can bring some relief to your body.

To make sure that we're getting adequate amounts of probiotics in our bodies to maintain our health, we must "refuel" with probiotic-rich food items frequently. An optimum diet full of probiotics may reduce or even reverse the effect of illness in our body.

Probiotics provide numerous benefits to our bodies and cannot be overlooked.

Probiotics & Gastrointestinal Function

Intestinal problems such as indigestion constipation, diarrhea and indigestion are extremely common and widely accepted as normal by the vast majority of us across the globe. A staggering 95 million American sufferers of Gastro Intestinal dysfunction. 2. It is around thirty percent of people. The Irritable Bowel Syndrome better known as IBS is among the top 10 reasons why you should see a physician within the United

States. Around $105 billion US dollars are paid for medical treatment of GI diseases within the United States every year.

The digestive system in our bodies is responsible for about 80percent of the overall immunity system's health. The improvement of your gut health has been demonstrated to improve your overall well-being and health.

Probiotics provide some of the most effective solutions for treating digestive health problems and perform a variety of particular things inside the stomach. Acidophilus and the other probiotics produce antifungal, antibacterial and antiviral compounds inside the intestine. Acidophilus is also responsible for creating an acidic microenvironment that helps in enhancing the absorption rate of iron as well as other minerals. Acidophilus also creates a layer or wall to stop the invading of bacterial and yeast.

The consumption of probiotic-rich food is proven to decrease symptoms associated with diarrhea, inflammatory bowel disease and food allergies. Certain studies are examining the harmful effects of probiotics on cancer of the colorectal. [3]

Probiotics, in essence, stop the growth of bacteria that cause harm in the gut, which set an increase in stress and inflammation during digestion. enhance absorption and digestion of trace minerals, such as calcium, and boost our overall metabolic rate.

Chapter 2: Probiotics & Your Immune System

The gut that is healthy typically filled with good bacteria. They are at war with unhealthy bacteria in your digestive tract. By feeding them regularly with probiotics foods boosts the allies, i.e. healthy bacteria who are able to protect your. In addition, boosting the healthful bacteria of the gut can strengthen around the 80% of your body's immune system's overall health.

It is a fact that we must all be aware of: the damaging micro-organisms that reside in our bodies. In our modern world, that a healthy diet aren't being practiced in sufficient amounts. Cheap, fast processed, sugary, food items that are genetically altered are all a click of a wrist. Many of them don't have any nutritional value that's healthy. In addition to sugars, preservatives, and carcinogenic ingredients in processed food The most hazardous substance in these foods is sugar.

The majority of the sugar in our diet is disguised by misleading labels. The words 'Fructose Sugar, Sweeteners as well as many others can be used to convince consumers into believing that foods aren't laden with sugar, when it is true that they're packed with sugar and can cause grave health problems for us. A variety of diseases are connected with a diet high in sugar. The development of diabetes is a clear result from a high intake of sugar. If the body is unable to further process sugar, it's converted to fat and stored in the body leading to weight gain. The cancer cells feed off sugar.

The bad bacteria living that reside in our guts flourish and grow rapidly whenever we consume foods that contain sugar. When they grow and begin outnumbering the beneficial bacteria the immune system, making us vulnerable to infection from disease. A natural solution to reverse this is to increase the amount of probiotic-rich foods to strengthen the immune system. Consuming probiotic-rich foods regularly will help you fight illnesses and maintain our health. Probiotics provide a natural defense mechanism for the body.

Probiotics & Brain Function

The mind, and our mood can be directly correlated with the health of our digestive system. The reason for this is that the greater portion of the serotonin that is that the brain uses is made in the stomach.

The state of health within our digestive system will influence how we use our brain, mood, and overall well-being. It is in fact the brain's second. If people talk about a gut sensation', they may actually be correct. The brain's interconnection with the organ systems of our bodies.

Probiotic bacteria have been proven to stimulate the development and growth of neurons. They also improve memory and learning, facilitate the changes that affect our mood, modify our digestion habits, and alter the way we express our genes. (Grossman, 2015)

Brain disorders caused by immune deficiencies and could lead to neuro problems. While the science of gut flora is a complex subject the researchers are engaged in a variety of studies that seek to discover the ways it could be helpful for treating conditions like Parkinson's, Alzheimer's as well as multiple sclerosis.

Other Health Benefits of Probiotics

In addition to digestive health, there are many additional benefits associated with taking probiotics. This includes:

They can reduce infection such as vaginal yeast and candida.

They can help manage blood pressure

They are able to help lower cholesterol levels.

This can aid those who are lactose intolerant digest lactose.

They are able to reduce the amount of the number of dental caries microbes that could exist in your mouth.

These help to fight allergic reactions.

They aid in lessening inflammation

These products aid in the rejuvenation of skin and also with particular skin disorders like eczema or dermatitis.

They aid in increasing metabolic rate and the natural flora of our body after taking prescription medications. [4]

Probiotics have numerous advantages that can't be adequately described as there's an ongoing research to learn more about these beneficial bacteria. It is not a mistake to consider expanding the number of these life-giving probiotics into our diet.

Chapter 3: Foods Rich In Probiotics

Many people use probiotic supplements. Even though nutritional supplements could provide positive effects, quantity and effectiveness of supplements containing probiotics is not certain. A research study conducted on 55 brands of probiotic products found that just 13% of these actually contained the amount of probiotics listed on the package. Furthermore, it's impossible to guarantee that the process of preservation won't harm the probiotics in the supplements. Probiotics are more fragile in comparison to other nutrients since they're alive i.e. 'living microorganisms'. These are most easily obtained from eating.

The majority of foods that contain probiotics are "cultures". These are foods that come from an initial food source that can be fermented so that you gain the benefits of probiotics in the final product. The process of fermenting food isn't an advanced method. The ancient days, food items were fermented in order in order to preserve them, or make a new dish or condiment out of them.

Fermentation breaks down components of food to the simplest form the bacteria convert carbohydrates into the acid lactic and yeast transform sugar to alcohol. Some people mistakenly think that probiotics can only be accessible through dairy products, but it is not true. There are other probiotic sources and they are ideal for lactose-intolerant people.

Whatever food item we select to consume to boost the amount of probiotics in our diet must be organic or organic. Many food preservation processes destroy probiotics. Beware of processed food, especially ones that have been pasteurized. They are not able to provide the required amount or quantity of probiotics. It's not difficult to find a item that will provide you with a nutritious dosage of probiotics regardless of which part of the world where you reside.

Here are a selection of the food items that are high in probiotics.

Live, Cultured Yogurt

Yogurt has always been regarded as the top food to consider when searching for an excellent supply of probiotics. The issue in yogurt is that the majority of processed yogurt available in the market is processed and is loaded with preservatives, sugars and sugars. as a result the yogurts do not have any probiotics whatsoever.

If you do choose to use healthier, organic products and non-sweetened types such as Greek yogurt, not all product is exactly identical. The higher-quality brands could have fewer probiotics, compared to ones that are perceived as less.

Unprocessed, organic, natural yogurts are the best choice for an adequate amount of probiotics. The sweetened, refined and packaged yogurts that are fancy don't have any substantial probiotic content or activity.

Yogurt made at home, without processing, has the highest amount of probiotics. Yogurt made with goat milk is thought to have the highest probiotic amount.

Knowing what to search for on a product's label is essential to find a product that is able to provide a sufficient quantity of probiotics. The labels that contain words such as "live and active culture" may have a greater amount of probiotics. A majority of yogurt manufacturers will also include the names of probiotics in the yogurt that it may have. It could include names such as bifidus regularis S.Thermophilus, bifidobacterium L.Bulgaricus and so on. [5] Verifying the label can help guarantee you that you will get the most the most value for budget. Beware of products that contain high levels of fructose levels, corn syrup, sugar, sweeteners, synthetic flavorings, additives and synthetic flavorings. The more simple, natural and free of flavor and the less likely it you will find a larger amount of probiotic.

Numerous research studies have been conducted, and it was found that the consumption of yogurt can be beneficial to digestion well-being (Irritable Bowel Syndrome [6] (IBS) as well as diarrhea) as well as upper respiratory diseases and even the health of the brain. There is only one condition: frequent and consistent consumption is needed before any major change can be detected.

Alongside probiotics, eating yogurt can provide a healthy amount of protein from animals along with other helpful nutrients such as vitamins and minerals. Individuals who have lactose intolerance may also enjoy yogurt.

Yogurt is delicious since it is a food that can be enjoyed with no further processing and in other foods such as such as desserts, smoothies, and other foods. If yogurt was cooked prior to use, the probiotics in it will be destroyed due to heating. It's best to consume it chilled or, at the very least, the temperature of room.

Kefir

Kefir (also called Keefir, or the word kephir) is enjoying a huge rise in the popularity of health food enthusiasts throughout the world due to many good reasons. Kefir is a drink that has been fermented that is made by adding kefir grain to cow or goat milk, and then allowing it to sit for 24 to 24 hours to begin the process of forming. The bacteria that live in Kefir seeds breakdown the lactose found in milk and convert it into the acid lactic. The milk is removed and the kefir grains with a gel appearance (which appear much like cauliflower) can be used again to make more Kefir. The milk that is strained tastes similar to the sour yogurt but is an adipose consistency.

The process of making kefir grains remains in mystery, with many theories and stories seeking to provide an explanation for the origins of these grains. At the time of their origin, they were believed to come by the gods. According to one theory, it was derived from the mouth of sheep, or bacteria in the intestines. A different version is that shepherds carrying milk inside bags made from leather observed that the milk would sometimes turn into an effervescent beverage. [7] Another story of the Caucasian mountains claims that the drink was given to them by Mohammed. Islamic Prophet Mohammed who walked his followers through the proper use of it and forbidden to reveal the recipe to anybody else, which is why they're often referred to as the 'grains from Prophet Mohammed'. Kefir's mystery of how it can be made is actually a blessing as scientists haven't found out the secret, making Kefir among the most genuine, unadulterated foods that exist that exists.

Kefir is not only full of nutrients, but it also offers a large number of probiotics. Kefir grains are a source of 30-35 different varieties of yeast as well as bacteria, which makes it more effective probiotic source than yogurt. Kefir is also a probiotic called lactobacillus kefir that is found only in kefir.

Kefir's biggest benefit is the fact that it's digested by people who have lactose intolerance [88.. In addition Kefir can be made in a variety of ways. Kefir can also be prepared by using non-dairy liquids, such as coconut water, or even fruit juice. An excellent tip is to prepare the drink yourself. It's very easy to prepare. Kefir that is sold in the market typically not long enough fermented and pasteurization has significantly decreased probiotics contained in the beverage. [9] Also, when making kefir make use of the grass-fed goats or cows' milk to ensure the highest supply of probiotics into the beverage.

Certain users recommend that you introduce kefir to your diet in smaller amounts and then increasing as time passes. If you consume large quantities at beginning can trigger undesirable reactions.

Miso

Since 2,500 years starting from the beginning of China up to Japan and even today miso has been a main ingredient. It's a tasty and delicious paste that is an ingredient in soups and has been said to provide antioxidant properties and neutralize the harmful effects of radiation, smoking as well as air pollution on your body.

The miso ingredient is a mixture or culture created by mixing cooked, ground soybeans, salt, koji and to create a smooth paste. It is later molded into balls before fermenting in a container up to six months or up to two to three months. [11] The more time miso ferments and the better quality of the final miso, in addition to having it being more rich, complex taste and aroma. Making miso is an art which has been refined through the Japanese.

It's important to define what koji means. Koji is often interpreted by non- Japanese as yeast, however it's actually a mold which has a sweet aroma and is made of rice cooked (12)which has been made with fermentation cultures commonly available in Japan also known as aspergillus Oryzae. Therefore, in a real way, koji functions as fermenting starter. Koji is utilized to make a variety of Japanese recipes including sake, soy sauce mirin, pickles, as well as rice vinegar.

Chapter 4: Sauerkraut

There are some people who have a tough digesting cabbage, and sauerkraut can be a fantastic alternative for those who struggle with it. Sauerkraut is also an excellent source of probiotics for those who have lactose intolerance to include probiotics into their food. Like many other food sources that contain probiotics Sauerkraut that is sold in the market place is typically preserved with pasteurization, which means it doesn't provide any nutrients from probiotics. Sauerkraut made at home is the best.

Sauerkraut simply means "sour cabbage"in German. It's a type of pickled cabbage that is made by cutting the cabbage, breaking it up and pressing or squeezeing the cabbage using salt [1414 for the purpose of extracting the juice or water, after which it is stored in a container filled with juice, which is then left to ferment over a period of 12 days or up to three weeks. If it's time to consume it changes in color between pale yellow and green.

Sauerkraut can be eaten chilled or hot, but if you wish to obtain probiotics from sauerkraut, it's recommended to consume it cold since heating destroys the probiotics. There are a variety of ways to consume sauerkraut cold meals. Some examples include toppings for hot dogs and sandwiches and including it in potatoes, cold salads egg dishes and fish or meat, or using it as a side dish to your main course. There are those who add sauerkraut to their vegetable smoothies. The sauerkraut juice by itself can be sold as a tonic for digestion.

The most significant nutritional benefit of sauerkraut is that it's an extremely abundant probiotic source. Sauerkraut really ranks high as a probiotic food source. The sauerkraut is believed to have the highest amount of probiotics in all dairy products and supplements available for sale. Research has been done to confirm this alarming information concerning sauerkraut.

The team that conducted the research that was led by probiotic fanatic Prof. Joseph M. Mercola discovered that a 4 to six ounce portion of sauerkraut had 10 trillion beneficial bacteria roughly approximately 100 times the number of bacteria found in the bottle of potent probiotics. [15] The results show that a 2 one ounce container of sauerkraut that has been fermented that you make at home provides roughly the same quantity of probiotics as 100 probiotic capsules. This means that it will take the equivalent of swallowing eight bottles probiotics in order to have the exact amount of nutrients inside a 16 ounce serving of sauerkraut that you make yourself!

As compared to yoghurt in this case, for instance, while 100 grams of yoghurt contain approximately 100 million components of probiotics. 100 grams of sauerkraut has a staggering 10, trillion pounds in probiotics! [16] "With every mouthful of sauerkraut, you're consuming billions of beneficial microbes which will be killing the pathogens in your gut driving them out and replenishing the beneficial flora in your digestive tract"According to According by Dr. Natasha Campbell-McBride during The 2013. The Gluten Summit. (Plotner, 2014).

Along with probiotics, sauerkraut is also a source of other nutrients, including Vitamin A and as much as 200x more Vitamin C over the cabbage's head. It is absolutely nothing to lose from eating this delicious nutritious food.

Microalgae (Spirulina & Chlorella)

Superfoods that thrive in the bottom of oceans are now becoming more popular due to of their capacity to enhance probiotics such as lactobacillus and Bifidobacteria within digestion. Some examples include chlorella, spirulina and the other blue-green algae edible. They are widespread throughout the world and are similar to bacteria but not seaweed.

They've been used to be a source of food for a long time and sometimes are available as powders. [17] [1818 A huge number of Asians, Olympic athletes and even NASA astronauts eat microalgae to get the full nutrition they provide. Spirulina has a 65% content of protein, and Chlorella contains 45% protein. Together, they provide other essential nutrients such as carbohydrate along with fiber, vitamins and minerals.

Spirulina is the most nutritious food source that is used for a long time. Apart from being nutrient-rich and nutrient-rich, it's also said to possess detoxifying qualities. Chlorella appears very much like the spirulina plant and has been proven to get rid of heavy metals within the body, and improve the health of your liver. [19] The high chlorophyll content will help detoxify the digestive tract. it also contains high amounts of antioxidants, protein and vitamins that are simple to take in. Also, they are loaded with energy, and boost your energy levels when taken in.

Recently it has become commonplace to introduce Chella and spirulina into fermented milk products like yogurt in order to enhance probiotic activity is becoming more popular. Microalgae like as these may increase the potential of probiotics present in dairy products that are fermented, such as yogurt.

One study demonstrated that the presence of spirulina and chlorella to fermented milk did not just increase the probiotic's viability in the milk, but also enhanced the function property of the probiotic well. (Beheshtipour, Mortazavian, Mohammadi, Sohrabvandi, & Khosravi-Darani 2013,) The reason for this is that both microalgae provide an array of Nutraceuticals and nutrients, hence they're "functional foods".

Functional foods are simply products that have health-giving ingredients.

Microalgae can be a rich source of powerful nutrition, There are a variety of ways to include them into your daily diet. According to research, the amounts of microalgae that are small tablets supplement (which may be about one teaspoon of powdered algae) is able to provide nutritional value of nutrients that are obtained from eating salads all throughout the day. You can add it in shakes, smoothies dairy, yoghurts and peanut butter sandwiches, or eaten in its entirety and taken in by drinking water.

Dark Chocolate

Raw, organic, and unprocessed dark chocolate offers many advantages for health and can be thought of as a food that is healthy. Mayans also considered cocoa to be"the food of the gods'. In the past, Aztecs ground cacao seeds, spices to make a drink that they believed would promote health, and they were accurate.

Dark chocolate is commonly considered to be a source of probiotics. However, it's in fact a fantastic natural protector for probiotics, so it can be a great addition to yogurt and other probiotic food items in order to protect the good bacteria they contain when they are consumed.

At Louisiana State University, researchers examined the effects the dark chocolate had on bacteria in your stomach testing three cocoa powders during a simulated human digestion process.20 The researchers found that gut's beneficial bacteria can process the flavonol-containing compounds found in dark chocolate, and reduce the fiber dietary found in the dark chocolate to ensure it's absorbed quickly.

The cocoa powder that is the basis of dark chocolate is produced is abundant in flavonol compounds, specifically epicatechin and catechin. Additionally, it is a source of fiber, which is converted. Gut bacteria that are good for you can break the polyphenolic polymers down into smaller anti-inflammatory compounds that can be quickly absorbed into the human body. [20]

In a more straightforward way the bacteria that live in our gut are capable of breaking down the nutrients of dark chocolate.

There are a variety of food items which contain probiotics. However, our stomach acids typically destroy these microorganisms before they reach the large intestinal tract. [21] The advantage that darker chocolates have over many of the probiotic food sources is that it delivers probiotics directly into the large intestinal tract without being damaged because of the acidity in the digestive tract's secretions. Dark chocolate functions as a natural defender against stomach acid and shields us from bio salts, which can destroy probiotics.

A study conducted at Ghent University in Belgium revealed that dark chocolate protects the probiotic bacteria that reside in the intestinal tract and stomach more effectively than dairy products such as yoghurt or milk. In the same study, researchers found there's three times higher chance that probiotics will survive in the presence of nutritious dark chocolate. (Possemiers , Marzorati , Verstraete, & Van de , 2010)

Chapter 5: Green Pickles

It is widely available and taken as a given, the typical pickle is an excellent food source for probiotics. Pickles are incredibly simple to prepare if you decide to not purchase the readily available commercial versions and they are delicious to eat.

Pickling food is not anything new or a novel method. It's been practiced since the beginning of time. In the year 2030BC, it's been recorded that cucumbers pickled originated from India in fact sparked a pickling tradition in Tigris Valley. It is believed that even Cleopatra knew about the advantages of eating pickles and was credited with her beautiful appearance to pickles. (Terebelsk and Ralph 2003) Pickles are a staple across many different cultures around all over the world. Whole cucumbers or even sliced cucumbers can be picked. Napoleon was so fond of pickles that he provided cash prizes to help find ways to keep their freshness for longer. This led to a man called Nicholas Appert to discover that submerging the glass jars for picking in a hot bath destroyed bacteria, and made the pickles to stay much longer. [23]

If you're purchasing and you aren't making your own pickle organic ones that don't contain vinegar and were made using no heat are the most effective alternative to obtain a high dosage of probiotics. Vinegar pickling i.e. placing the vegetable's greens in acetic acid and vinegar significantly slows the development of pathogenic microbes as well as yeast that are present in pickles.

Most of the time, the majority of pickles sold in the market is made using vinegar, as making pickles with vinegar prolongs the shelf-life of the item more. There are exceptions, however. half-sour varieties typically produced in brine with no vinegar, and stored in grocery stores that sell health foods. They tend to be more expensive than when they make by hand.

homemade pickles that are fermented with water along with spices and brine is most delicious. If you put greens in a jar inside the kitchen and mix in salt, water and spices, the vegetables produce their own lactic acid that keeps the vegetables. The acids themselves are an inevitable byproduct of fermentation. This method is the traditional way of making pickles without vinegar and it is known as 'lacto-fermentation'. The sugars from greens soaked in brine bind onto the outside and exchange with lactic acid bacteria. They make lactic that creates the unique taste and allows it to remain usable for longer periods of time. As with most fermented food items, pickles contain a lot of probiotics.

The shorter fermentation times of a few weeks generally result in pickles that are half-sour while longer fermentation times led to lighter-colored pickles, with a more tart taste.

Pickles can be consumed by themselves as snacks, or as a sandwich ingredient hotdogs, hamburgers, hotdogs or salads. Because pickles can be consumed cold, you're guaranteed to be consuming the probiotics in them whenever you consume pickles.

Kombucha

It tea is an Asian fermented tea, which has been consumed for centuries and contains probiotics. There are numerous evidences of the potency of this tea. It's believed to increase immunity, assist in weight loss, improve metabolic rate of the body, assist in the detoxification process and ease joint pain.

Kombucha is thought to originate from China and then spread around the globe to gain its current popularity among those who advocate healthy food. The legend says that the Japanese King, Inyko, was healed by the Korean medical practitioner known as Kombu who offered the tea. Cha is Chinese which means tea. Therefore, it is a mixture of the words 'Kombu' and 'cha' gives the tea its current name.

Sometimes referred to as an "immortal wellness elixir', it is believed to provide an energy boost and improve your immune system, enhance sleep, excellent for acid reflux among other things. It is crucial that you make your own kombucha at home, that it is done in extremely clean environment.

Kombucha is created through mixing tea black an organism of bacteria as well as yeast, referred to as Scoby (24) along with sugar and of the kombucha inside a glass container, such as the jar. It is then allowed to ferment over a period of 7-12 days to reach 30 days. The longer the kombucha has been fermented, the more bitter it turns because the sugar in it is disintegrated. This is the reason why many drinkers add juice to their older drinks that are sour so that the flavor is easier to tolerate.

The health-conscious should be aware that the sugar found in the kombucha drink isn't to be avoided since it's what scoby 'eats to break down and generate probiotics. A different trend in recent times is to replace regular coffee with decaffeinated to decrease the caffeine content of kombucha.

Kombucha is a rich source of nutrients that help to regulate the metabolism of your body so that it naturally heals it self, which is the reason many people believe that it can cure many ailments.

The thing you should be aware of about the kombucha drink is that it can create a worse situation before making you better. One way to think about it is the fact that bad bacteria within your body are able to block any good bacteria brought to it. Kombucha isn't for everyone initially, and it could cause more symptoms for certain ailments before finally giving some relief. Start with small doses to assist in decreasing the severity of this problem.

As well, women in pregnancy and children aged 10 and under, as well as those who are using blood thinners should not to drink Kombucha. A minimum of 4-8 bottles a day are recommended.

Tempeh

Tempeh is made of whole soybeans whose the husks have been removed, after that, they are cooked in part and followed by mash and fermentation with mold. In the process of fermentation, the mold is able to break down the mashed soy and then binds the molecules to form the form of a cake. Tempeh is a popular choice for vegans and vegetarians to alternative to bacon, meat or tofu.

Its ancestry is thought to originate originally from Indonesia many centuries back. Today, it is consumed all over the world. Tempeh originates from solely soya beans is very popular in Indonesia. And in other regions around the globe, the soya bean that is used to make tempeh can also be mixed with millet, and barley.

The fermentation process that tempeh experiences allows it to be digested and absorb. It is a delicious savoury and slightly nutty flavor that are described as earthy and sweet.

It's an ideal probiotic food. It is a rich source of beneficial microorganisms and bacteria, especially Rhizopus Oligosporus 2525. which improves our digestive health, and consequently the body in general. The fungus or mold that ferments tempeh produces naturally-produced antibiotics [26(26, 27) that help counteract the harmful adverse effects of bad bacteria within the body.

Furthermore, it's abundant in other nutrients such as vitamin and protein along with minerals like manganese and iron as well as others trace minerals. The plant-based protein is comparable to the animal protein.

Although tempeh that is sold in stores can be convenient however, it's likely to be processed, meaning it may lack the probiotic bacteria that can be useful to your. The ones that are sold in the commercial market usually possess a slightly bitter finish.

The process of making yourself your own tempeh [27It is a good idea however, you must take some time to master the art of controlling temperatures during the process of fermentation. But once you've been able to master the process the next steps will appear to be a breeze. It is also guaranteed that you will be able to get the probiotics that you require in your own homemade recipe.

Tempeh is prepared in many methods. Tempeh can be cooked and fried or even cooked. In Indonesia it is offered at almost every local market as well as in villages. It can be cooked and then served in soups or rice. It is also on the menus of most upscale restaurants. Also, it is great to serve as a barbecue food or stir-fried and served as a sandwich topping alternative. Tempeh patties are used in place of beef used in hamburgers. Tempeh is also commonly used for Asian sauces. Tempeh can be served as raw food, though the taste of the raw tempeh may not please everyone.

Kimchi

A lot of times, it is used as a side dish to many dishes, such as dumplings, soup, rice and rolls. Especially in Korea and Japan, Asian fermented cabbage could be best described as a more spicy and slightly sour-tasting variant of sauerkraut.

Simply put, cabbage is immersed in brine in order to eliminate all harmful bacteria in it. Then it is then soaked in a spice mix called gochugaru[28] and let to ferment for 1 to 5 days. Some of the most delicious Kimchi is the one which are allowed to ferment for around two weeks.

In this time the process of lacto-fermentation takes place. Lactobacillus bacteria breakdown the sugars present in cabbage, resulting in lactic acid that leaves the cabbage with an unusual bitter taste. Kimchi that has been fermented is most effective preserved in the fridge.

Kimchi has a significant amount of probiotics i.e. beneficial bacteria strains. According to some sources, about 12 lactobacillus strains that thrive in duodenum and stomach are present in the kimchi. Additionally there are probiotic strains found in kimchi are able to stick to the gut better than the probiotics found in supplements (Lee and et al. (2010)).

Chapter 6: Aged Cheese

In recent times, cheese has received lots of bad press, specifically for excessive cholesterol levels and for promoting overweight. It is however easy to forget that some individuals, similar to the French have been eating cheese greater than the majority of us and are healthier and have fewer cases of heart disease than Americans.

Research conducted from researchers from the American Chemical Society showed that in addition to balancing the intake of saturated fats, exercising actions, eating a variety of veggies and fruits, were additional things that the French took care of that improved their overall health. Quantity and quality of cheese that we consume can also be a factor. The consumption of cheese with moderation is essential, as is choosing the best cheese brands. (Bushak, 2015)

Two or three ounces of cheese per day is an acceptable amount to maintain. Choose natural fermented cheese in lieu of brands that have been that are injected with bacteria from the producer is recommended. The highest quality cheese to provide high quantities of probiotics is cheese composed of unpasteurized, raw milk from cow or goat as well as cheese that is aged. However, cheese that has organic or'made with raw milk', or "probiotic" on the label is the most reliable choice.

Naturally fermented cheese is brimming of lactic acid bacteria, which benefit the overall health. It is in fact fermented milk curds, and the types of starter bacteria utilized along with the process and duration of the fermentation process are specific to different varieties of cheese. This is why different kinds of cheese contain different kinds of the lactic acid bacteria.

The low acidity of cheese and its high fat preserve make cheese the best mediums through where healthy bacteria can thrive and also be transported around within the digestive tract, without becoming damaged.

The most common rule regarding cheese is that every type of cheese could contain probiotics so it is not cooked or pasteurized following the time they're made. However, it is true that cheese can provide healthy probiotics to the body only if it's not cooked prior to being consumed.

Types of Cheese

Cheddars like Colby cheese, Monterey Jack, Cottage cheese

Lactococcus lactis subsp lactis

Lactococcus lactis subsp cremoris

Streptococcus thermophilus

Italian Cheeses such as Parmesan, Romano, Provolone and Mozzarella

Streptococcus thermophilus

Lactobacillus delbrueckii subsp bulgaricus
Lactobacillus helveticus

Lactobacillus lactis

Different types of cheese, including Brick, Limburger and Muenster

Lactococcus lactis subsp lactis

Lactococcus lactis subsp cremoris

Streptococcus thermophilus

Lactococcus lactis subsp biovar diacetylactis

Lactobacillus delbrueckii subsp bulgaricus
Lactobacillus lactis

Lactobacillus casei subsp casei

Cheeses with "eyes" such as Swiss, Emmental, Gouda and Edam

Lactococcus lactis subsp lactis

Lactococcus lactis subsp cremoris

Streptococcus thermophilus

Lactobacillus delbrueckii subsp bulgaricus

Lactobacillus lactis

Lactococcus lactis subsp biovar diacetylactis

Leuconostoc mesenteroides subsp cremoris

Propionibacterium shermanii

The cheese that has been mold-ripened includes Brie, Camembert, Blue, Gorgonzola and Stilton

Lactococcus lactis subsp lactis

Lactococcus lactis subsp cremoris

Lactococcus lactis subsp biovar diacetylactis

Leuconostoc mesenteroides subsp cremoris

Goat Cheese

Lactococcus lactis subsp lactis

Lactococcus lactis subsp cremoris

Lactococcus lactis subsp biovar diacetylactis

Leuconostoc mesenteroides subsp cremoris Culled from Probiotics-LoveThatBug.com (Rotarangi, Different Types of Cheese and the Lactic Acid Bacteria in Cheese)

Sheep Cheese

Lactococcus lactis subsp lactis

Lactococcus lactis subsp cremoris

Lactococcus lactis subsp biovar diacetylactis

Leuconostoc mesenteroides subsp cremoris

6 Other Probiotic Foods

The list of foods that have probiotics doesn't end with the 11 that have been discussed. There are many more however, we'll discuss six additional probiotic food items below.

Chapter 7: Wheat Grass

The majority of sprouted seeds and grains are very nutritious. Wheatgrass comes from seeds. They contain a substantial amount of chlorophyll as well as fiber. Chlorophyll in combination with fiber can help improve colon health and is essential for probiotics to flourish and help us stay healthy. To extract the best nutrition of wheatgrass, the seeds can be dried or juiced and grinded into a powder and blended into smoothies and shakes.

Buttermilk

Buttermilk is the natural byproduct of the butter-making process. As milk is processed, it is separated into two parts that are butter and Whey. Whey is what is known as buttermilk. If it's made by hand the whey will usually be filled with naturally-occurring bacteria called lactic acid that helped make the milk ferment before it's turned into a churn. It is a delicious acidic flavour that can be beneficial in the preparation of many dishes particularly pancakes, pastries pudding, or even to substitute for yoghurt in recipes. But, in order to reap maximum benefit from the health bacteria that it has the milk should be consumed chilled or served as a cold dish such as desserts, salads and even in a dish that is served as a complement to the main course. The buttermilk you buy from the store is typically processed and is usually skimmed milk that culture has been incorporated into. Traditional buttermilk purchased at health food stores is ideal and should be sure it's organic and state on the label the presence of live cultures.

Sourdough Bread

This is a specific type of bread that is made using an initial starter which is then fermented over a period of at least 1 day, or longer before being mixed with additional ingredients to form bread. It is the result of fermentation that produces an sourdough starter with an abundance of probiotics.

Due to this, many people think that sourdough is high in probiotics also. One of the problems with this assertion is that the majority of bacteria be killed by the heat needed for baking bread. Probiotic claims found in bread sourdough may require additional study.

Beer

The readily available, commercially-priced beers we drink each day aren't always probiotic, even though they are produced by an alcoholic process however, the yeasts as well as live bacteria that are present in them tend to be destroyed at the conclusion of the manufacturing process once they're pasteurized. The more dark, non-filtered and unpasteurized and higher priced varieties of beer typically have living cultures. However, they must be consumed with moderation in order to reap any health benefits. They generally have a higher alcohol percentages [3131 similar to wine, they may age due to their living cultures.

Their flavor gets better with maturing, and the alcohol content increases as the wine ages.

Natto

It is a stringy fermented soybean Japanese food that has a distinct spicy smell and distinct taste. It's rich in probiotics and bacillus subtilis, which was which was previously referred to as bacillus antito. Natto and rice are the most popular breakfast item in Japan however it's being included in sushi, salads and even in burritos. Natto is a fantastic source of protein from plants as well as a source of Vitamin K. Sometimes natto is served with sweet sauce that contains a lot of fructose. A healthier option to consume Natto is to avoid the sauce altogether and choose soy sauce.

Non-Dairy Probiotic Food Sources

Probiotic-rich food items appear to be the most popular groups. They can be found in dairy products, or fermented plants or grain. The prevalence of lactose intolerance is increasing. issue across the globe, however it doesn't mean anyone with lactose intolerance has a disadvantage in the field of the probiotic food options. There are a variety of options that you can choose from.

Fermented foods made from vegetables such as sauerkraut, pickles and even Kimchi are excellent alternatives for those who are lactose-intolerant. Foods that are fermented with soy beans like miso and tempeh are also fantastic alternatives for dairy. Thus, lactose intolerance really isn't significant.

As mentioned several times throughout this book the process of fermentation is actually responsible for breaking down the complicated compounds found in food, and can make it easier for humans to absorb and digest. This is true for all foods, including dairy-based. Kefir, a dairy product, is an ideal illustration. Although kefir is a dairy-based, the introduction of kefir grain into milk, and the process of fermentation that it goes through to make the kefir beverage breaks lactose to produce an result that can be accepted by those who have lactose intolerance.

The best aged and hard cheese that has lower liquid content can be consumed by people who are lactose-intolerant since the reason for its hardness comes in the absence of lactose, which is a liquid. Try to include the probiotics you need in a sufficient amount in your daily diet, even if you're lactose-intolerant.

Chapter 8: Comparison of Bacteria

The babies are born with a small amount of bacteria that reside in the stomach. In some ways, the digestive tract acts as the blank canvas that is preparing it self to absorb data. Therefore, in the mother's womb the gut of an infant is almost sterile. The fetus's gut is still to acquire the diverse species of bacterial species that constitute the microbiome an person will have throughout his or her life. When a baby leaves mother billions of bacteria begin entering and expanding into this new home. Hundreds of billions will be able to settle at their new place of residence in the baby's gut. The tiny community that grows and evolves over the coming months, days and years, which scientists are discovering, could have a major impact on your future health.

An article in The Journal of American Medical Association (JAMA) of the infant's digestive tract can go a long way to explain what takes place within the first couple of weeks or days of a baby's life. Researchers took stool samples of more than 102 infants who were full term, the with an average gestational period of nearly 40 weeks. The babies were being born to women from New Hampshire when the babies were just 6 weeks old. which is the age chosen as eating patterns tend to be set by this time. Based on telephone interviews

* 70 of the infants were exclusively nursing (never getting any form of formula)

Formula * 6 received exclusively

* 26 consumed a mix of breast milk and formula.

According to medical records, 70 babies were delivered vaginally, while 32 babies were born through Cesarean births. Researchers also inquired about (non-topical) medication that infants received prior to birth. Also excluded from the study were infants that had been treated with antibiotics (antibiotics remove the gut tract biome, causing the bacteria in the gut have to be introduced back into the gut).

Then they analyzed each set of associations--feeding method and delivery method--separately. If they controlled for the food method, researchers observed significant variations in the composition of baby's intestinal bacteria, compared to those who were born by cesarean or vaginally. A different bacterial type was observed based on technique of feeding. That is breast vs. formula.

If they were able to control for the delivery method, exclusively formula-fed babies had a microbiome that was distinct from those of others. The combination-fed infants had the same digestive compositions as infants only formula-fed (though they did not gather data on the proportion of breastmilk and formula for the combination-fed group).

Differentialities between Gut Bacteria based on Delivery

The colonization process of the Babies stomach was different depending on the birth. What are some variations? Bacteroides was the largest genus of bacteria that was found within about 25% of newborns. It was being followed by Bifidobacterium within just one quarter.

* Bacteroides species made up 35% of vaginally-born infants' guts, and 21% of cesarean birth baby's guts. It was responsible for 28% of breast-fed exclusively babies' guts as opposed 22% for combo fed along with 29% formula fed infants"guts.

* Bifidobacterium was found to be 23% of vaginally-born infant's guts. It also made up 17% of the cesarean birth infants"guts," 26% of breast-fed exclusively infants' guts one-third of the combination fed infants' guts as well as 11% of infants fed formula"guts".

The proportions of the eight different genus of bacteria, which included Streptococcus,

Clostridium, Lactobacillus and Staphylococcus -- were not as significant as were the bacteria that were more prevalent overall. However, the differences were evident.

So What Do These Differences Mean?

These findings revealed variations in gut bacteria which are statistically significant. The question to be determined is if these changes are clinically relevant.

The latest study suggests that breastfeeding can contribute to the formation of healthy bacteria within the gut of a newborn. Researchers found that 3 months-old infants who were exclusively breastmilk-fed had greater diversity of bacteria that resided in their stomachs as compared to babies who were fed just formula.

Researchers also discovered an association between the microbes in infants' digestive tract and the variations in the expression patterns of the genes with their immune systems.

Research is revealing that the first neonatal stage is crucial in the development of intestinal digestion and also colonization of the gut by bacteria.

Breast-Fed vs Formula

This study focuses on the differing concentrations of bacteria in the gut that live within the gastrointestinal tract based on food choices, including breast milk as opposed to. formula in the initial several months of the being born. This study found an association but not an causal link breastfeeding and a better gut for infants, but it is necessary to verify the results.

However, there is a way to explain in a plausible manner why breast milk could cause changes to a infant's gut bacteria as well as the immune system. Researchers concluded that "The greater diversity of bacteria seen in the guts of the breast-fed infants may bring about the activation of certain immunity genes." (See Resources #1)

Breast Milk Vs. Formula

In a different study, scientists searched for genetic information in the stool of 12 babies -- the majority of which were breast-fed as well as the remaining half were formula fed. Researchers used genetic information to determine the kinds of bacteria that resided in infants the guts of their babies.

Chapter 9: Breastfeeding

The American Academy of Pediatrics (AAP) advises breastfeeding as the most nutritious food for babies. Baby should be exclusively breastfed throughout the first six months, says the AAP. When other food options have been added in the meantime, the AAP advises mothers nursing until their infant is at minimum a year old. They also recommend breastfeeding until the mother and baby will.

Breastmilk is beneficial for babies in a variety of ways.

The natural antibodies can help protect your child from diseases, including an ear infection.

It's typically easier to digest than formula. Thus, babies who are breastfed tend to be less gassy and constipated. This can reduce the chance of sudden infant deaths syndrome within the beginning of your child's life.

This can boost the intelligence of your child. The research shows that infants who breastfeed are more cognitively active. functioning. Breastmilk may also aid your child later on as it reduces the likelihood of being overweight, as well as in the event of developing asthma types 1 and 2 diabetics, high cholesterol leukemia, Hodgkin's Disease, and lymphoma.

The benefits of breastfeeding are good for mothers also. Breastfeeding mothers have lower risk of developing breast cancer, diabetes osteoporosis and heart disease and Ovarian cancer. The main reason breastfeeding mothers choose to do so is. It's a great bonding time with your child. (See Resources #3)

Friendly Vs. Unfriendly Gut Bacteria

Healthy bacteria assist in the metabolism of nutrients. They also aid in the process of helping certain chemicals enter the bloodstream. An array of healthy flora helps protect the intestinal tract from less beneficial kinds.

However, an overwhelming quantity of unbeneficial floraand that can be triggered by eating a diet that is high in sugar, fat and processed foods could cause stomach discomfort, gas in the stomach, and bloating as well as inflammation. "The flora can also emit chemicals that compromise the intestinal lining" According to Lita Proctor of the Human Microbiome Project at the National Institutes of Health. "This so-called 'leaky gut' allows nonnutritive materials to slip into our bodies and affect how we feel."

It's amazing that some bacteria can actually cause weight gain. The twins studied in a recent study which was published in Nature revealed that when the bacteria of the obese human twin were in the digestive systems of slim mice, mice became fat. In the event that bacteria from the thinner twin were introduced to mice that were lean, the mice were able to maintain their weight. Research suggests that diabetes and obese sufferers have a lower diversity of bacteria. The Cleveland Clinic found that some bacteria can metabolize egg components and animal meats to create an ingredient that assists in clogging arteries.

"This might explain why some unhealthy eaters get heart disease while others don't," Hazen explains. Hazen.

There's good news that it is possible to change the gut bacteria in your body and swap bad bacteria with healthy ones.

"Get the right type in your gut and, depending on your condition, you may begin to see improvements in a matter of days or weeks," claims Edmond Huang, a metabolic biologist at the University of California, Berkeley.

In order to cultivate a healthy microflora you must feed those species that are desirable while taking away the undesirable ones. Take care with antibiotics that destroy the microflora that keeps our bodies fit and healthy, along with the ones that cause illness and infections.

"Every course of antibiotics has a chance for such complications as yeast infections, skin rashes, and allergic reactions," claims Liponis.

Take these medicines only in the event of need, and add probiotics in order to replenish the beneficial living flora.

Probiotics

In the World Health Organization (WHO) 2001 defined the term "probiotics" to be "live micro-organisms which, when administered in adequate amounts, confer a health benefit on the host".

While there are a myriad of claims for benefits to using commercial probiotics, for instance alleviating stomach pain or improving the immunity. A systematic study of 15 human controlled randomized research studies conducted in July of 2016 showed that certain strains available in the market of probiotic bacteria belonging to the Bifidobacterium and Lactobacillus genera, when consumed through mouth daily in doses of between 109-1010 colony-forming units (CFU) for about a month enhanced the performance of people suffering from specific psychological disorders, e.g. depression, anxiety and autism spectrum disorders and obsessive-compulsive disorder. They also increased specific elements of memory.

Probiotics for Brain Health

Five probiotic species that support the health of your brain are:

1.) Lactobacillus Plantarum remain in your stomach for an extended period and can help control immunity and manage inflammation within the gut. A good source is kimchi as well as sauerkraut.

2.) Lactobacillus acidophilus is a good supplement to in boosting the immune system, by keeping the balance between healthy and harmful bacteria at bay. The best sources of this are dairy fermented items like yogurt and kefir.

3) Lactobacillus brevis - helps improve immune function. The best part is that it's been proven to boost levels of brain-growth hormone (BDNF) that is brain derived neurotrophic factor. It can also be beneficial to consume this strain while using antibiotics since it can aid to maintain the health of your microbiome. A good source of sauerkraut is pickles.

4.) Bifidobacterium lactis - helps to prevent digestion problems and increase the immune system. It's found in products made from fermented milk, such as yogurt.

Chapter 10: Choose Food-Based Probiotics First

Probiotics, the beneficial bacteria that are found in fermented foods as well as supplements -- boost the quantity of friendly bacteria that live in your gut. If you're relatively healthy It's a great plan to start by eating authentic food first before consuming supplements.

Bifidobacteria is a common ingredient in yogurts, produce chemical compounds that produce an acidic atmosphere in which numerous harmful bacteria cannot thrive. The yogurt that contains the standard variety Lactobacillus rhamnosus can enhance your mood. A study from 2013 published in Gastroenterology showed that healthy women who consumed two servings of 125g of yogurt every day for four weeks the brain scans of their subjects showed less of a response confronted with negative images.

Feeding Your Microbiota

This is a list of foods that are good to ferment to consider eating regularly live-cultured yogurt Kefir and kimchi, kombucha tea sauerkraut, pickles fruit and vegetable pickles.

Also, you should cut down on sugar consumption as well as increase the amount of dietary fiber you consume. In addition, if you're taking probiotics, it's important to consume prebiotics (explained in a later post) so that the healthy gut bacteria to grow and thrive in your gut.

So What is a Probiotic?

Probiotics are microorganisms considered to offer the health benefits of eating. Probiotics are currently utilized to refer to ingested microorganisms that have benefits for humans as well as animals. Probiotics came into popular usage after the year 1980. The concept's introduction is usually attributable to Nobel laureate Elie Metchnikoff. He proposed that yogurt drinkers Bulgarian farmers lived longer as a result of this practice. In 1907, he suggested the idea that "the dependence of the intestinal microbes on the food makes it possible to adopt measures to modify the flora in our bodies and to replace the harmful microbes by useful microbes". An exponential growth in the probiotic market has raised the need to establish scientific proof of the positive effects of microorganisms.

Elie Metchnikoff first suggested the possibility of colonizing the gut with beneficial bacteria at the beginning of the 20th century.

Another Reason to Use Probiotics

Recent research with mice indicates that probiotic supplements could slow the loss of bone following menopausal change. Mice showed hormone changes that are similar to those seen with menopausal women. Following the intake of probiotics every week for a month, the mice retained their bone mass. The group who was not given probiotics reduced by 50% their bone volume during this period. The mice ate Lactobacillus that was found in yogurt, along with eight different strains of probiotic bacteria.

Eat Plenty of Prebiotics

If you're not familiar about the concept of "prebiotic", these are substances that stimulate the development or activities of microorganisms (e.g. bacteria, viruses and fungi) which contribute to the wellbeing of their host. One of the most popular examples is in the gastrointestinal tract which is where prebiotics modify the composition of microorganisms that make up the microbiome of your gut. Prebiotics possess three characteristics 3 characteristics: 1.) Incompletely digestible, they aren't disintegrated through gastric acids or enzymes found in stomachs.

2.) They need to be capable of being fermented or processed by intestinal bacteria.

3.) It must be beneficial for the patient - like what effect food fibers have on the development of healthy bacteria within the digestive tract.

To further elaborate on feature #1 of a diet plan, prebiotics tend to be non-digestible substances that are absorbed by the upper portion of the gastrointestinal tract. They increase the activity or growth of beneficial bacteria which colonize the bowel's large intestine by serving as a substrate. The first time they were identified and categorized in the work of Marcel Roberfroid in 1995.

Function

The definition of prebiotics does not emphasize any specific category of bacterial. In general the assumption is that prebiotics will increase the activity or number of bifidobacteria as well as the lactic acid bacteria. The value of the bacteria bifidobacteria, as well as lactic acid bacteria is because the bacteria in these two groups could provide numerous benefits to the human host, particularly regarding digestion (including increasing the absorption of mineral) as well as the efficacy and strength intrinsic to our immune system. An item that promotes bacteria that bifidobacteria are considered to be a bif element.

Health Benefits of Prebiotics

1.) They help reduce the severity of fever-related illnesses caused by diarrhea or respiratory incidents.

2.) They decrease inflammation in digestive disorders and help can help prevent colon cancer.

3.) They improve absorption of minerals within the body, such as calcium and magnesium (which may cause an rise in the density of bones).

4.) They may reduce the risks of developing cardiovascular disease in decreasing inflammation.

5.) They may help prevent weight gain (their effects on hormones that are related to appetite) through the production of lower levels of ghrelin which is the body's signal for the brain that it's the time to take a bite.

6) They lower the amount of glycation. Glycation can increase free radicals, creating inflammation and weakening the intestinal liner.

Top 10 Foods Containing Prebiotics

Although there isn't a general agreement on the ideal daily intake of prebiotics guidelines typically are between 4 and eight grams (0.14-0.28oz) for general digestion health, and up and up to fifteen grams (0.53oz) and more, especially for individuals with active digestive problems. Based on an average 6g (0.21oz) daily serving here are the prebiotic amounts in ingredients needed to get the daily requirement of prebiotic fiber.

The foods mentioned above have insoluble fiber that could be utilized through "Prebiotic" bacteria and subsequently let their nutrients out for use in the body of the person.

The use of prebiotics is effective in reducing infections that require antibiotics, and the quantity of illnesses in infants aged between 0 and 24 months.

Research has shown that prebiotics increase production of short-chain acid fatty acids (SCFA) but more study is required to prove the causal link. Prebiotics could be beneficial for the inflammatory bowel or Crohn's disease by generating SCFA to nourish colon wall, as well as reducing ulcerative colitis-related symptoms.

In the immediate aftermath, the addition of large levels of prebiotics into the diet can lead to an increase:

* Fermentation that leads to an increase in gas production as well as bloating and intestinal movement.

* The production of SCFA and the quality of fermentation is reduced in long-term eating regimens with low fiber intake.

In the meantime, until bacterial flora becomes created to restore or repair the intestinal microbiome, absorption of nutrients could be compromised and it is possible that the colonic transit times may increase temporarily when you add more prebiotics. (See Resources #4)

Chapter 11: Enteric Nervous System

The enteric nervous or the intrinsic nervous system, is one the principal divisions of autonomic nervous system. It consists of a mesh-like network of nerve cells that regulate the functioning of the gastrointestinal system.

Structure

The nervous system of the enteric nerve consists of approximately 500 million neurons. This is two-hundredths of the total number of neurons found in the brain. That's more than five times the hundred million neurons found in the spinal cord. This is approximately 2/3 of the total nervous system in the cat. The system for the nervous system in the enteric region is embedded within the lining of our gastrointestinal system. It starts with the esophagus before all the way to the anus.

The Enteric nervous system (ENS) or the intrinsic nervous system is among the major divisions of the nervous system. It consists of a set of neuronal networks that control the functions of the digestive system. The ENS is often considered to be distinct from the autonomic system because it operates on its own action.

The ENS can perform independent functions, such as co-ordination of reflexes while it also receives a significant amount of input through the autonomic nerve system. However, it is able to perform its functions independently from the brain and spinal cord.

Like all body systems, the ENS function may be affected due to Ischemia (cell dying).

The system of the enteric nervous system is identified as the "second brain" for several reasons. The system of the enteric nervous system is able to be autonomous. It usually communicates with Central Nervous System (CNS) via its parasympathetic (e.g. through the Vagus nerve) as well as sympathetic (e.g. through the prevertebral Ganglia) nerve systems. Yet, research in vertebrate anatomy shows that if you cut off the Vagus nerve is damaged then the system that controls the enteric nerve remains in operation.

In vertebrates, the intestinal nervous system can carry reflexes, and also serving as an integrator without CNS input. Sensory neurons provide information about physical and chemical factors. In the intestinal muscles, motor neurons manage peristalsis and production of intestinal contents.

Others control the release of various enzymes. The nervous system in the enteric tract utilizes thirty neurotransmitters, the majority of them are similar to those in the CNS like dopamine, acetylcholine and serotonin. Over 90% of our serotonin is located within the intestines, as and around 50percent of our body's dopamine. Dopamine is currently being researched for further understanding its role in brain function.

The nervous system of the enteric tract can alter the way it responds based on things as the amount of food and composition. Furthermore, ENS contains support cells that are like the astroglia in the brain as well as there is a diffusion barrier in the capillaries around ganglia that is similar to the blood brain wall of blood vessels in the cerebral cortex.

The Gut Brain

The gut is a brain that is its own. It's it's the system of enteric nerves. Like the bigger brain inside the head scientists say that this brain transmits and receives signals as well as records the experiences of others and reacts to emotional responses. The nerve cells in the system are influenced and bathed by similar neurotransmitters. Gut disorders can affect the brain, just like it can cause brain damage. stomach.

The brain of the gut, also known as the "enteric nervous system" is found in the sheaths the tissue that lines the esophagus small and large intestines as well as the colon. It is thought of as a singular entity. it's made up comprised of neurons, neurotransmitters as well as proteins that transmit messages between the neurons, as well as support cells that resemble neurons that are found in the brain as well as a complicated circuitry that allows it to function independently to learn, recall in addition to, as the phrase is, create gut-feelings.

The brain of the gut is believed to play an essential part in human happiness as well as sadness. Numerous digestive diseases like colitis, irritable bowel syndrome and others result from issues within the brain of the digestive tract. It is also recognized that the majority of cases of ulcers originate from microorganism, not because of anger towards one's mother.

Details of how the enteric nervous system mirrors the central nervous system have been emerging in recent years, according to Dr. Michael Gershon, professor of anatomy and cell biology at Columbia-Presbyterian Medical Center in New York. He is one of the founders of a new field of medicine called "neurogastroenterology."

People suffering from Parkinson's or Alzheimer's conditions are afflicted by constipation. The gut nerves function just as neurons in their brains. Similar to how the central brain influences the gut, the brain of the gut has the ability to relay information back to the brain. A majority of the feelings that come into conscious awareness include negative ones such as gas and pain.

The ENS image (This system is maintained throughout into the Gut). Notice the Mysenteric plexus as well as the Submucous plexus.

Myenteric plexus lies between the circular and longitudinal layers of muscle that form the tunica muscularis. It correctly, is responsible for exerting control on the digestive tract's motility.

Submucous plexus like its name suggests it is located beneath the submucosa. Its primary function is understanding the environmental conditions within the lumen, controlling gastrointestinal blood flow, and regulating epithelial cell functions. When the functions of these cells are not as important like the esophagus and the submucous plexus appears to be sparse, and could be absent within sections.

Apart from the two main enteric nerve plexuses there are a few minor plexuses below the serosa and within the smooth circular muscle, and within the mucosa.

Inside the plexuses in the intestine there are three kinds of neurons that are primarily multipolar.

Sensory neurons are able to receive signals via sensory receptors within the mucosa and muscles. There are at least five distinct sensors have been found within the mucosa that respond to heat, mechanical or chemical stimulation. Chemoreceptors that respond to acid as well as amino acids have been identified that, is what allows "tasting" of lumenal contents. The muscle's sensory receptors react to tension and stretch. Together, the sensory neurons in the enteric tract make up a large database of data on the contents of your gut as well as the condition of the wall in the gastrointestinal tract.

Motor neurons located in the enteric plexuses regulate gastrointestinal motility, the secretion process, as well as absorption. While performing these roles motor neurons work directly on an array of effector cells. These include smooth muscles and secretory cells (chief mucous, parietal and the pancreatic exocrine cell) as well as gastrointestinal endocrine cell.

Interneurons are responsible for the integration of sensory information and transferring the information to ("programming") motor neurons.

Enteric neurons release a range of neurotransmitters. The most important neurotransmitter released by these neurons is Acetylcholine. The majority of the neurons that produce acetylcholine tend to be excitation-driven, triggering muscles that contract, increases the secretions from the intestinal tract, and production of hormones in the enteric tract as well as dilation of blood vessels. Norepinephrine is used in a variety of ways to transmit neurotransmitters in the digestive tract, however it comes from extrinsic sympathic nerves. Norepinephrine's effects are nearly always inhibiting and in opposition to the effect of acetylcholine.

The nervous system in the digestive tract can be autonomous however, normal digestion requires the use of communication channels between the system's intrinsic components as well as the central nervous system. These connections take the form of sympathetic and parasympathetic nerves that link the enteric and central nervous systems, or link the central nerve system to digestion. By means of these connections it is possible for the gut to transmit sensory signals to the CNS and also the CNS could affect the functioning of the digestive system. The connection to the central nerve system can also mean that signals that originate outside the digestive system could be transmitted to the digestion system. In other words, the visual of food that is appealing stimulates the production of secretions within the stomach.

Chapter 12: Digestive Enzymes

The enteric Nervous System is responsible for controlling a large portion of the digestive process. There are four major places where digestive enzymes are produced, which are:

* Salivary glands

* Secretory cells located in the stomach

* Secretory cells located in the pancreas

* Secretory glands within the small in the intestine

Enzymes are special proteins created to degrade a specific food chemical. Release of enzymes may tie in to the control of hormones. The enzymes are classified according upon the type of food they operate with (Substrate):

* Peptases and proteases split proteins into small peptides as well as amino acids.

The lipases divide fat into three fat acids and the glycerol molecules.

Amylases are enzymes that break down carbohydrates like sugars and starch into simpler sugars like glucose.

Nucleases break down nucleic acids and nucleotides.

The digestion system of the human body, the principal areas of digestion include:

* The Oral cavity

* The stomach

* The small colon

Digestive enzymes are produced by various exocrine glands that are located in the mouth, stomach the small intestine as well as in the pancreas.

Mouth

The complex food ingredients that are consumed need to be broken down into simpler dissolvable, soluble and palatable substances prior to their being taken in. The mouth cavity is where salivary glands release a variety of substances and enzymes that assist in digestion as well as cleaning. The following are some of them:

Lipase Lingual: The process of digestion begins within the mouth. Lingual lipase begins the process of digestion of lipids or fats.

* Salivary Amylase The digestion of carbohydrates can also begin through the mouth. Amylase, which is produced by salivary glands, dissolves complex carbohydrates into smaller chains, or simple sugars. Sometimes, it is known as ptyalin.

* Lysozyme: In the event the fact that food is far more than the essential nutrients, e.g. viruses or bacteria, the lysozome serves a limited, not-specific but beneficial antiseptic effect in digestion.

Stomach

The digestive enzymes produced within the stomach are referred to as gastric enzymes. The stomach is a key function in digestion as a matter of fact through the mixing and crushing of food and in an enzymatic way in that it digests the food. There are a variety of substances, hormones or enzymes generated by the stomach and the function they play:

Pepsin is the principal gastric enzyme. It is made by stomach cells known as "chief cells" in its inactive form called pepsinogen. The pepsinogen enzyme is activated by stomach acid, transforming into the active form of pepsin. Pepsin reduces the proteins in food into smaller fragments that include amino acids as well as peptide fragments. The digestion of proteins begins within the stomach. This is different from the digestion of carbohydrates and lipids which begin their digestion through the mouth.

Hydrochloric acid (HCl) It is essentially positively charged hydrogen atoms (H+)

which is also known as stomach acid. It's made by the cells of the stomach known as parietal cell. HCl is primarily used to destroy the protein ingested to remove any bacteria or viruses which remains in food and to convert pepsinogen into.

Insic factor (IF) Insic factor is created by parietal stomach cells. Vitamin B12 is a crucial vitamin that needs support to ensure absorption by the an ileum that is terminal.

mucin. The stomach is an obligation to eliminate organisms and viruses that reside in the acidic environment it has, but is also required to safeguard its lining against the acid. The method by which the stomach does this is through producing bicarbonate and mucin through the mucous cells in addition to the rapid turnover of cells.

Gastrin is a vital hormone created in stomach cells "G cells" of the stomach. The G cells release gastrin as a reaction to the stretching of stomach that occurs when food is introduced into the stomach as well as after exposure to proteins. Gastrin is an endocrine hormonal hormone that is why it gets into the bloodstream, and then returns to the stomach. It stimulates parietal cells and produces the acid hydrochloric (HCl) as well as Intrinsic factors (IF).

Gastric Lipase: This is a lipase that's acidic produced by the gastric chief cell within the mucosa fundic of the stomach. Its pH is optimum between 3 to 6. The gastric lipase, along with tongue lipase, are two lipases that are acidic. They, like alkaline lipases (such like pancreatic lipase) are not dependent on the use of bile acids to ensure optimal enzyme performance. Acidic lipases comprise 30 percent of the digestion-related lipid hydrolysis in humans and gastric lipase supplying to the largest proportion of both acidic lipases.

There are four kinds of stomach cells:

Parietal cells produce the chemical hydrochloric acid as well as intrinsic factor.

Chief cells of the gastric tract produce pepsinogen. Chief cells can be found within the stomach's body that is located in the superior or middle anatomic part of the stomach.

Pit cells and mucous neck produce bicarbonate and mucin in order to form an "neutral zone" to protect stomach linings from acids or irritations that can occur in the stomach chyme.

G cells create gastrin, a hormone in response to the distention of stomach mucosa or proteins and also stimulate parietal cell producing their secretion. G cells are found within the inferior part of the stomach.

Chapter 13: Pancreas

Pancreas is an endocrine and exocrine gland. This is because it produces endocrinic hormones which are released into circulation system (such as insulin and glucose) in order to regulate sugar metabolism and for the production of digestive juice or exocrinic that is then released through the pancreatic tube into the duodenum. The exocrine or digestive function of the pancreas is just as important for maintaining good the health of the body as its endocrine functions.

Two cells found in the pancreatic parenchyma comprise the digestive enzymes that it produces:

Ductal cells: primarily responsible for the production of bicarbonate (HCO3) and works to reduce the acidity of stomach chyme that enters the into the duodenum via the pylorus. The pancreas' ductal cells are activated by the hormone secretin for the production of bicarbonate-rich bile that are an in essence a biofeedback system Highly acidic stomach chyme entering duodenum causes the duodenal cell called "S cells" to produce secretin hormone and release into the bloodstream. The secretin that has entered blood ultimately comes in contact with the pancreatic ductal cell, activating them to create bicarbonate-rich liquid. It's important to remember that secretin can also block the gastrin's production from "G cells", and is also able to stimulate acinar cells within the pancreas, which produce pancreatic enzyme.

Acinar cells: primarily involved in the production of Pancreatic enzymes that are inactive (zymogens) which, after being found in the small bowel, activate and play a major role in digestion by breaking down proteins DNA/RNA, and fat. Acinar cells are stimulated by cholecystokinin (CCK), which is a hormone/neurotransmitter produced by the intestinal cells (I cells) in the duodenum.

CCK boosts the production of pancreatic Zymogens.

Pancreatic juice, which is made up of the secretions produced by both ductal as well as acinar cells, is composed of digestive enzymes such as:

Trypsinogen is a non-active protease, is activated by the duodenum to form trypsin, disintegrates proteins into amino acids. Trypsinogen is activated through the enterokinase duodenal enzyme to form its active form, trypsin.

Chymotrypsinogen It can be described as an inactive protease is activated when enterokinase duodenal, transforms into chymotrypsin and is able to break down proteins in their amino acids that are aromatic. Chymotrypsinogen can be also activated through trypsin.

Carboxypeptidase, an enzyme that removes the amino acid group at the end from proteins. A variety of elastases degrade proteins elastin as well as other proteins.

Pancreatic lipase degrades triglycerides to fatty acids as well as the glycerol.

A variety of nucleases which reduce nucleic acids like DNAase as well as RNAase.

Pancreatic amylase is able to break down glycogen and starch and glycogen, which are polymers of glucose that have an alpha linkage. Humans aren't equipped with cellulases (enzymes) that digest carbohydrates cellulose that is a beta-linked glucose molecule.

Exocrine pancreas function is owed a part of its flawless function to biofeedback mechanisms that regulate the release of the juice. The following bio-feedback pancreatic mechanisms are crucial in maintaining the the balance and production of pancreatic juices:

Secretin, the hormone created by duodenal "S cells" in response to the stomach chyme that has an extremely high concentration of hydrogen atoms (high acidity) releases in the blood stream after returning back to the stomach secretion reduces gastric emptying and enhances pancreatic ductal cells and also stimulates the pancreatic acinar cells in releasing their enzyme-producing juice.

Cholecystokinin (CCK) is an exclusive protein released by the duodenal "I cells" in response to chymes that have significant protein or fat content. In contrast to secretin which is an endocrine hormonal hormone, CCK is actually a stimulator of the neuronal system and the result is the stimulation of the acinar cell to let their contents out. CCK can also increase the contraction of the gallbladder which results in the squeeze of bile through the cystic drain, the common bile duct, and finally the duodenum. Bile is a natural ingredient that aids in the to absorb fats through emulsifying it and increasing the absorption surface. Bile is produced by the liver, however it is stored within the gallbladder. GIP, a gastric inhibitory protein (GIP) is created by mucosal duodenal cells when chyme is stimulated. It contains significant amounts of carbohydrate proteins, fat acids. The primary function of GIP is to slow down the rate of emptying gastric juices.

Somatostatin is a hormonal substance that is produced by mucosal cells from the duodenum, and those of the "delta cells" of the pancreas. Somatostatin is a powerful inhibitory impact, including the pancreatic enzyme production.

Small intestine

The following hormones and enzymes are made by the duodenum

Secretin: It hormone is produced by duodenal "S cells" in response to the acidity of gastric chyme.

Cholecystokinin (CCK) is an exclusive chemical released by duodenal "I cells" in response to chyme that has proteins or fats with high levels. Contrary to secretin, an endocrine hormonal hormone, CCK is actually a stimulator of a neuronal network that's end result is the stimulation of acinar cells that let their contents out. CCK additionally increases the rate of contraction in the gallbladder and causes the release of stored bile through the cystic duct which then flows into the common bile drain and through the ampulla of Vater to the second anatomic location in the duodenum. CCK reduces the strength of the sphincter Oddi, the sphincter responsible for controlling flow in the ampulla of Vater. CCK reduces the activity of gastric cells and reduces the rate of gastric emptying thus allowing the pancreatic juices in order to neutralize the acidity in the gastric the chyme.

Gastric inhibitory Peptide (GIP) This protein reduces gastric motility. is made by the duodenal mucosal cell.

Motilin: The substance improves the motility of the gastro-intestinal tract through specialized receptors referred to as "motilin receptors."

Somatostatin is a hormone created by the duodenal mucosa as well as it is also produced by pancreas' delta cells. It's principal purpose is to block the secretory mechanism of a number of.

Within the lining of small intestine, there are a variety of brush border enzymes that's purpose is to break down the chyme that is released by stomach into digestible particles. These enzymes can comprise:

Erepsin converts peptones as well as polypeptides to amino acids.

Maltose converts maltose to glucose.

Lactase: It is a vital enzyme that transforms lactose to galactose and glucose. Most Middle Eastern and Asian populations are deficient in this enzyme. It also declines as you the advancing age. This is why lactose intolerance frequently a frequent abdominal problem in Middle Eastern, Asian, and older people, manifesting as constipation, abdominal pain as well as osmotic diarrhea.

Chapter 14: The Probiotic Planet

Just like a planet, the healthy human body is home to massive amounts of probiotic kinds that are beneficial to our overall health. It is estimated that there are around ten percent more probiotics in our bodies than our cells. Consider this carefully.

The body is more microbial that cellular. Probiotic bacteria comprise around 70 percent in our immunity. Researchers are even suggesting that the probiotic's DNA may be greater than our cells' DNA when it comes to forecasting our vulnerability and potential new diseases.

One hundred trillion probiotics live within a healthy digestive system, roughly 3.5 pounds. The digestive tract is home to around 400 to 500 different species of bacteria. Twenty species comprise around 75% of all the species but there are others.

A lot of them are native strains that are attached to the intestinal wall. A few are transitory. They usually last for less than two weeks.

Most of our probiotics are found in the colon however, billions of them also reside within our mouths and the small intestinal tracts. There are other populations of bacteria as well as yeasts reside in our skin, beneath toe nails, within the vagina, between our toes and within all the other body nooks and cavities. Sometime, they reside in regions including joints as well as other internal tissues.

Microbial Realization

Western medical science was unaware that there was a bacteria before 1673 when Dutch researcher Antony van Leeuwenhoek began writing letters to the Royal Society of London about the pictures he had seen through his microscope, which he had invented.

in 1674 Leeuwenhoek described the bacteria he observed in the nearby lake. The writer wrote that the bacteria were "wound serpent-wise and orderly arranged, after the manner of the copper or tin worms." In 1683, he wrote about the his findings of bacteria from the dental plaque. He talked about "many very little living animalcules."

Bacteria research continued with a fascinating manner up to the point that some scientists such as Edward Jenner, Ignaz Semmelweis, Friedrich Henle and Louis Pasteur believed that diseases are mostly caused by microorganisms.

The connection between disease and germs isn't an original one, but. Before Leeuwenhoek even saw his "animalcules," ancient medical experts had proposed that numerous illnesses are caused by small microbes. The ancient medicine of the time contemplated the invasion of the forces of disease, and there were even vaccines.

The renowned Middle Eastern physician Avicenna discussed the spread of infectious diseases in his 1020 A.D. Canon of Medicine. Italian doctor Fracastorius believed that syphilis and Typhus are caused by infectious microbes. Many thousands of years before, Ayurvedic medical science identified the presence of cells that are infected within the pathologies of disease.

Western medical research discovered that there was a connection to the immune system as well as these immune cells in 1796 in 1796, when the doctor. Edward Jenner scraped smallpox blisters off of a person who had contracted cowpox while milking cows. The pus was gathered on a piece of wood, and then was injected into the arms the boy who was eight years old. Another 23 people were also injected following the boy had survived. The lower incidence of smallpox in the group of people who were injected was evident as the current method of vaccination came into existence.

Microorganisms and Disease

We are becoming more aware that microorganisms are the cause of numerous ailments. Although we have tried to disinfect the workplace and our home and workplaces, we continue to be sick by microorganisms.

Why do we live in clean, disinfectant-treated homes and clean our hands with soaps that are antibacterial yet we still contract many infections from microorganisms?

In the present, despite our numerous antibiotics and disinfectants, as well as antivirals oral rinses and antiseptic cleaning products Infectious diseases have been on the rise. The incidence of tuberculosis and influenza or shingles, mononucleosis malaria, cytomegalovirus HIV, AIDS and herpes have been increasing across the world.

It has been estimated that about a third of the people living in the first world might be suffering from Herpes Simplex 1, while thousands of million are suffering from the genital variant, Herpes Simplex 2. Over half of the globe's population is infected with Helicobacter pylori. A large portion of all over the globe are suffering from sexually transmitted illnesses like the syphilis, gonorrhea or chlamydi.

It is reported that the World Health Organization said over 34 million people in the world had been diagnosed with HIV during 2010, an increase by more than 16% annually over the last two years. Within the U.S. alone, there around 40,000 instances of HIV recorded each year.

Around one-third of the population in the world is affected by the tuberculosis bacteria. In a year, 6 million suffer from TB as per the U.S. Centers of Disease Control. More than a million people are afflicted with illnesses that are transmitted by water around the globe.

The majority of these ailments and a variety of others have a direct connection to infectious microorganisms through the use of bacteria viruses, fungi or bacteria. You might be shocked by some of the illnesses microorganisms have been linked to. Look at the following table:

Strange diseases connected with microorganisms

Disease

Some Suspected Microbes

Cardiovascular diseases and stroke

Helicobacter. Pylori

Treponema pallidum (syphilis)

Staphylococcus aureus

Enterococci faecalis

Streptococcus species

Herpes Simplex (I and II)

Pneumonococcal aerogenes

Candida albicans

Streptococcus mutans

Escherichia coli

Chlamydia pneumonia

Porphyromonas gingivalis

Tannerella forsynthensis

Prevotella intermedia

Gallstones

Eubacteria

Clostridium species

Ulcers,

ulcerative colitis as well as

Crohn's

Helicobacter Pylori

Clostridium species

E. coli

Mycobacterium pneumoniae

Cancers

Staphylococcus aureus

Enterococci faecalis

Streptococcus species

Pneumonococcal aerogenes

Streptococcus mutans

E. coli

Mammary tumor virus

papilloma virus (HPV)

H. Pylori

Heptitis B

Diabetes

Coxackle B virus

Cytomegalovirus

Salmonella osteomyelitis

Others are suspected (see arthritis in the next section)

Arthritis

Bacteroides fragilis

Borrelia burgdorferi

Brucella melitensis

Brucellae species

Campylobacter jejuni

Chlamydia trachomatis

Clostridium difficile

Corynebacterium striatum

Pyarthrosis caused by Cryptococcal

Gardnerella vaginalis

Kingella kingae

Listeria monocytogenes

Moraxella canis

Mycobacterium lepromatosis

Mycobacterium marinum

Mycobacterium terrae

Mycoplasma mycoplasma arthritidis

Mycoplasma hominis

Mycoplasma leachii sp.

Neisseria gonorrhoeae

Ochrobactrum anthropi

Pasteurella multocida

Pneumocystis jiroveci

Porphyromonas gingivalis

Prevotella bivia

Prevotella intermedia

Prevotella loescheii

Pseudomonas aeruginosa

Pyoderma gangrenosum

Roseomonas gilardii

Salmonella entertidis

Scedosporium prolificans

Serratia fonticola

Sphingomonas paucimobilis

Staphylococcus aureus

Staphylococcus lugdunensis

Streptococcus Agalactiae

Streptococcus equisimilis

Streptococcus pneumoniae

Streptococcus pyogenes

Streptococcus uberis

Tannerella forsynthensis

Treponema pallidum

Vibrio vulnificus

Yersinia enterocolitica

Alzheimer's disease

Chlamydia pneumoniae

Borna virus

H. Pylori

Spirochetes

Herpes simplex I

Picornavirus

The overgrowth of yeasts such as Candida albicans are also known to cause or be the major cause of a variety different diseases. Studies have revealed that, in certain instances, Candida albicans can grow in conjunction with Staphylococcus Aureus, which can cause the rapid development of both. It can lead to various diseases that are due to the combination of yeast and bacteria. The bacteria and viruses can be able to grow together. It is seen in a lot cases of deaths caused by influenza swine flu as well as other. The majority of deaths occur among people who have been immunosuppressed, and also suffer from concurrent bacteria infection.

Types of Microbes

Fungi

Molds, yeasts and other more than 100,000 species are found in air, earth or water as well as humid and humid environments. They can be transmitted to the body through the air, food and the your skin

Bacteria

Single-celled organisms that live in earth, water as well as in air. They also live within living organisms may be infected through food, water and the the skin

Viruses

Non-living, genetic mutation triggers that occur in water the air, earth and skin Infects by altering the cellular DNA and then spreading throughout continuous cell division and change

Mycoplasmas

Slow-moving ancient bacteria that thrive on the water and earth; they typically infect through the touch of water, food or even through contact

Parasites

tiny organisms that are infected and reside within a living organism. This includes protozoa, worms, and amoeba

Thermophiles

Opportunistic bacteria which can be found in extreme hot environments for example, hot deserts, boiling water, and even ovens

Psychophiles

Opportunistic bacteria which can be found in extreme cold temperatures like the artic, or even within freezers.

Nanobacteria

Very small bacteria which usually possess a calcium-based hard shell. It is believed that they cause conditions that are thought to be auto-immune.

Presently, we face numerous infections resulting from the various types of microorganisms. The most prevalent infectious diseases on the list are lyme disease (Borrelia Burgdorferi) as well as pneumonia Staphylococcus and streptococcus the salmonella, E. coli, Listeria, cholera and shigellia. Dengue fever yellow fever and tuberculosis. Cryptosporidiosis is also a concern, as Hepatitis, rabies, and many more. A lot of these microorganisms are increasing despite antibiotics and antiviral medicines. Many are growing due to intoxic sex, contaminated waters, or changes in the land's use.

The Rise of the Superbugs

The number of infections is increasing as a result of opportunities that arise due to our devastation of the environment. A lot of others are developing resistance to the antibiotics we use. They are commonly called superbugs.

One of the more dangerous of these superbugs is methicillin-resistant Staphylococcus aureus (MRSA). MRSA prevalence is increasing as nearly every institution--the most important jewels in the antimicrobial world--is infected MRSA. A 2007 study from one hundred and twenty-one U.S. hospitals, 46 of the 1,000 patients admitted to hospitals are infected or colonized by MRSA and 75 percent of them affected.

The potential virulence of Staphylococcus aureus was first discovered around 1929, by

Alexander Fleming, a microbiologist who cultivated a mixture of Staphylococcus aureus in conjunction with an expanding mold. He observed the penicillin-producing mold eliminate certain bacteria, but other bacteria, but not all. Fleming discovered that Staphylococcus aureus quickly adapted to penicillin. It then became resistant. In the present, Staphylococcus aureus is still one of the best resistant to antibiotics.

Staphylococcus aureus is also considered to be one of the lethal bacteria that has been identified to date. It releases three toxins to kill cells that include alpha toxin, beta toxin, and leukocidin. They all bind cells' membranes and break them down that allow cytoplasm and the contents of cells to escape. The result is that the cell dies. the cells. The immune system has problems tackling and eliminating Staphylococcus aureus since it produces enzymes that counteract the immune system's defense strategies. Staphylococcus aureus can adapt very rapidly and the more you put it through is the stronger it will become.

Infectious bacteria may not be identified in all diseases. In recent years, we have been discovering that a variety of common illnesses have been caused or exacerbated through fungal or bacteria-related diseases. There is also an increase in the number of chronic diseases that are caused by infection, including arthritis, heart disease ulcers, IBS, asthma as well as chronic fatigue syndrome.

The Oral Bacteria

Don't forget about the microorganisms in the gums and teeth. Numerous pathogenic microorganisms may develop and thrive in the dental, gums and mouth. This includes:

* Streptococcus mutans

* Streptococcus pyogenes

* Porphyromonas gingivalis

* Tannerella forsynthensis

* Prevotella.

A few of these microbes thrive in roots canals. They provide safe spaces to allow bacterial growth. The bacteria that infect the root canals be a mix of steptococci staphylococci and potentially dangerous spirochetes including Borrelia burgdorferi and many more. Any bacteria that may infect the body may hibernate within the canals of the roots.

Since root canals are encased as well as the surrounding tissues are dying their surrounding tissues, the immune system can't access these locations to eradicate the bacteria. In the end, many diseases are being linked with roots canal-harbored bacteria.

Chapter 15: Our Anti-Microbial Society

The seemingly endless growth of infections and microorganisms persists despite the use of prescription and prescription antibiotics, antifungals, and antivirals as well as antiseptic soaps disinfectants for cleaning has exploded in the last few years.

The importance of microbes in the fight against disease is reflected by both authorities of the government and parents around the globe. Microbes are seen as a threat number one by U.S. Centers for Disease Control as well as government anti-terrorism officers and the respective agencies across other nations. The concern over microorganism-related outbreaks and pandemics has placed microbes prominently on the pages of a variety of newspapers as well as newscasts.

However using antibiotics has risen dramatically in the last few years. Nowadays, 3 million pounds of natural antibiotics are used by humans every year throughout the United States alone. Then there's the about 25 million pounds of antibiotics that are given to animals every year.

However, a lot of antibiotics are either given for a lack of efficacy or ineffectiveness. According to the Centers for Disease Control states that "Almost half of patients with upper respiratory tract infections in the U.S. still receive antibiotics from their doctor." However, the CDC cautions that "90 percent of all upper respiratory illnesses, which includes children's ears infections, are caused by viruses which means that antibiotics aren't able to help viral infections. About 40 percent of the 50 million antibiotic prescriptions every year from doctors office were ineffective."

In fact, the increasing use of antibiotics is also creating the Pandora's Box of superbugs. When bacteria are hit repeatedly by the same antibiotics that they adapt to, they develop. Like any living thing can do (yes bacteria exist) bacteria are taught to ward off and fight against frequently used antibiotics. This is why a lot of bacteria are today resistant to various antibiotics. It is due to the fact that bacteria tend to change their environment. If they're afflicted enough repeatedly by a specific problem, they will eventually be able to determine how to avoid the challenge and prosper in spite of it.

The same is true with a variety of emerging antibiotic-resistant strains. The bacteria have evolved and be stronger and better able to take on these strategies.

This has led to the creation of multiple-drug resistant organisms (MDROs). The most dangerous MDROs include those from Enterococcus, Staphylococcus, Salmonella, Campylobacter, Escherichia coli as well as other. Superbugs, such as MRSA are also classified as MDROs because the majority of MRSA cases have been found to be resistant to a variety of antibiotics.

Another advancing MDRO strain can be identified as Clostridium difficile. The bacterium can infect the intestinal tracts of anyone of any vârstă. For children, this is among the world's largest killers, with acute and diarrhoea that is watery. Also, it is an increasing illness among adult. Each year, C. difficile is a source of infection for the tens of thousands across the U.S. according to the Mayo Clinic. More importantly, C. difficile are more and more resistant to antibiotics, and infections due to clostridia are increasing with each passing year.

Summary of Common Antibiotics

Type

Examples

Use and Side Effects

Penicillins

Amoxicillin

Ampicillin

Azlocillin

Carbenicillin

Cloxacillin

Dicloxacillin

Flucloxacillin

Mexlocillin

Meticillin

Nafcillin

Oxacillin

Penicillin

Piperacillin

Stapholococcus species, Streptoccoccus species, STDs, E. coli,

Lyme disease, and others

Skin itching, allergic reactions, anaphylactic reaction and kidney damage. injury, brain damage and probiotic loss

Macrolides

Azithromycin

Clarithromycin

Dirithromycin

Erythromycin

Roxithromycin

Troleandomycin

Telithromycin

Spectinomycin

Pneumonia Streptococcus species mycoplasma infections, Lyme and many more.

The adverse side effects of jaundice include as well as liver damage, nausea, vomiting, diarrhea as well as skin rashes and the probiotic death-off

Aminoglycosides

Amikacin

Gentamicin

Kanamycin

Neomycin

Netilmicin

Streptomycin

Tobramycin

Paromomycin

Gram-negative bacteria, such as E. coli, Klebsiella and Pseudomonas.

The adverse side effects of this medication are skin rashes and kidney damage, loss of hearing vertigo and destroying the probiotic systems of your body.

Glycopeptides

Teicoplanin

Vancomycin

Gram-positive bacteria

Similar side effects to those mentioned previously mentioned

Polypeptides

Bacitracin

Colistin

Polymyxin

Gram-positive bacteria

A topical agent, or inhaled.

Allergic reactions and the elimination of probiotics

Carbapenems

Ertapenem

Cilastatin

Doripenem

Imipenem

Meropenem

Broad spectrum (gram-positive and negative)

The adverse side effects of this include

seizures, headaches, rash, allergies, nausea and probiotic die-off

Quinolones

Ciprofloxacin

Enoxacin

Gatifloxacin

Levofloxacin

Moxifloxacin

Norfloxacin

Ofloxacin

Pneumonia UTIs, STDs, others

The adverse side effects of this include

Neuropathy in the peripheral region, tendon tear, damaged nerves, damage to the liver and the depletion of probiotic colonies.

Tetracyclines

Demeclocycline

Doxycycline

Minocycline

Monocycline

Oxytetracycline

Tetracycline

STDs such as mycoplasmas and acne, malaria Lyme disease, and many more

Negative effects may include GI damage and liver damage. Other adverse effects include the stunting of growth, tooth staining as well as fetal toxicity and probiotic death.

Sulfonamides

Co-trimoxazole Mafenide

Sulfacetamide

Sulfadiazine

Sulfamethizole

Sulfasalazine

Trimethoprim

Sulfamethoxazole

Burns, UTIs, dermatitis and acne, as well as fungi other

Side effects that can be harmful include the kidneys failing, reduced white cells counts, renal crystals itching, nausea, vomiting, and destroying the our probiotic system.

Cephalosporins

Cefadroxil

Cefazolin

Cefalexin

Cefaclor

Cefproxil

Cefoxitin

Cefdinir

Cefditoren

Cefotxaxime

Cefepime

Ceftobiprole

Broad spectrum

Adverse side effects include skin rashes, nausea, seizures, headaches, diarrhea, and eliminating

Probiotic colonies.

Chloamphenicol

Chloamphenicol

Broad spectrum

The adverse effects of anemia and probiotic loss

Clindamycin

Clindamycin

Broad spectrum, acne

Clostridium, Pseudomonas, etc.

Other adverse reactions include vomiting, diarrhea, colitis and cramps. They also can cause rash and contact dermatitis as well as probiotic die-off

Lincomycin

Lincomycin

Similar to Clindamycin

Ethambutol

Ethambutol

Tuberculosis and other diseases;

Affects adverse: damaged nerves and color blindness. Probiotic death

Metronidazole

Metronidazole

Guillaminosis, vaginosis and giardia and nausea, stomatitis or leucopenia, black tongue Nerve and probiotic death-off

Rifampicin

Rafampicin

Gram-positive, mycobacterium

Acute reactions include rashes and tears coloring. Probiotics die off

The reason why there are numerous antibiotics available is the same reason why some pathogens are getting intolerant to many of our antibiotics. These are strategies that remain static that are not a part of the living system. Living systems can be adaptive. They adapt to everything that comes their way. Furthermore, each of the antibiotics we've created is effective in preventing microorganisms using the same method each time. Certain antibiotics will block the wall of the microorganism's cells.

Other will affect the cell's RNA--at the very least, until they adjust.

How Bacteria Become Antibiotic Resistant

Over time, microorganisms is able to learn how to deal with almost every threat to its existence. To protect it and its colonies the microorganisms will slowly discover ways to avoid threats. Through the course of many generations this strategy is learned and refined through successive generations of bacteria.

For a better understanding of how bacteria develop resistant to infection, imagine an intruder broke into a residence when the family was at home. The homeowner is armed with a baseball bat. He strikes the burglar in the head. The burglar flees. One month later, the burglar enters the home again. What would you imagine the thief will be wearing this next time? Of course, a helmet!

It is important to understand that all bacteria, even pathogenic bacteria are living organisms who are simply trying to survive. Thus, when they face an overwhelming threat, such as an antibiotic, in the span of generations they'll find out a way to get against that antibiotic. This is accomplished through the introduction of subtle gradual changes to their gene.

There is a possibility that bacteria can spread antibiotic resistance. It's interesting to note that bacteria aren't the only ones to produce a genetic variant they also produce an extremely small and compact package of genetic material called a plasmid that they are able to transmit their gene-related variation to different bacteria.

The plasmid can also be described as Replicon because it could be passed to another bacterium that will then incorporate the genetic data into their own. The new bacterium is able to replicate exactly the methods of the original bacterium. When it is inside the organism, the plasmid allows bacteria to use the antibiotic's workaround as well as transfer the plasmid to an additional bacteria.

Our antibiotics with broad spectrum could be thought of as a baseball bat, in the metaphor previously mentioned. When used, bacteria can change to this static (antibiotic) device. Many species may find an alternative to the antibiotic.

After being learned, the trick becomes a cloned technique that is then passed on to the other kinds of bacteria. And in the near future, antibiotics will become ineffective against a variety of species. The ability to acquire knowledge from a different species level offers one of the most terrifying aspects concerning bacteria: the capability of different species to increase beyond our capacity to eradicate the bacteria. The ability to combat the static antibiotics we use isn't just about resistance. It is also about resilience.

While bacteria travel across humans, animals trains, buses as well as airplanes, they will keep acquiring resistant to antibiotics. The result will be many of our antibiotics becoming ineffective.

Why Probiotics Provide the Solution

Probiotics can solve this dilemma. What is the reason? Probiotics are intelligent living organisms. They are also the most feared foes of these pathogenic species.

Actually, our probiotics as well as nature's pathogenic bacteria have been fighting for millions of years and probiotics are beating the pathogenic bacteria! The proof is provided in the reality that humanity's race continues to exist. It means that the probiotics are able to detect the newest plasmids, and then respond with their individual strategies and plasmids that fight pathogenic bacteria.

As in our analogy of burglaries, once the burglar is back with his helmet on when he returns, the person in the home pulls out a different weapon in order to frighten the criminal. If the burglar is with the right weapon in hand then the homeowner will come up with an alternative.

For a better understanding of how efficient and effective probiotic bacteria can be in the production of antimicrobial substances, researchers in the Department of Microbiology of the Abaseheb Garware College in India looked into the genus of Steptomyces as early as the 1970s. They found that it was making new antibiotic compounds exponentially through time. The researchers graphed logistically the number of antimicrobial chemicals produced through time, and concluded that the genus has the capacity to produce more than 100,000 antibiotic compounds!

Living organisms do to defend their territory. When probiotic and pathogenic bacteria compete each one is developing innovative strategies to fight one another. If one of them develops a novel method, the other create a different one. The two throw their own naturally created antibiotics at one another and each reacts with a similar response.

Probiotics have been proven to possess the same instruments at their disposal. Probiotics can also develop antibiotic resistance just as pathogenic bacteria like MRSA (antibiotic-resistant staph) can.

Researchers of the Swedish University of Agricultural Sciences found that, not just could Lactobacillus reuteri probiotic strain easily acquire resistance to antibiotics: L. reuteri also developed the plasmids. The researchers found L. reuteri carrying two plasmids that have created and passed through antibiotic resistance two antibiotics, lincosamide and tetracycline.

The Invasion

Many different kinds of microbes may be found within the food we eat. Clostrium botulinum is a common occurrence in the juice or food containers particularly cans which can cause fatal illness known as botulism. Campylobacter is among the most prevalent bacteria found in food, and is usually present in animal products. The result is vomiting, fever and cramps however, it is not always fatal.

The E. Coli bacteria could occasionally cause death in immune suppressed individuals, however for the majority of people, it can cause a bit of nausea, and sometimes a couple of days of diarrhoea. Salmonella can be found within the intestines of a variety of animals, including reptiles, birds and various creatures (including people). The virus can also result in a mild nausea or diarrhea in a normally healthy individual.

In spite of the fact that warm and humid places are the most desirable but bacteria can also survive in extreme conditions. They're able to live in fridges, in freezer, and even low oxygen vacuum bottles. At lower temperatures, the bacteria are able to be incubating.

Just a bit of warm water can revitalize billions of bacteria and trigger colonies. Many foodborne bacteria colonize via the release of spores, which can survive even the harshest conditions--including pasteurization. A single spore may expand into an entire population of bacterial colonies.

Pasteurization

We believe that we're fighting off bacteria by using the arsenal of antimicrobial protections we have. Our bleaching, antibacterial soaps, and floors that have been disinfected will protect us from these germs.

Many of us are prone to an illusion of security when it comes to our processed foods. We believe that, since most producers pasteurize their food products and ensure that they are free of bacteria. However, this is not the case.

French chemical engineer Louis Pasteur developed pasteurization in the 1850s in order to debunk the idea of spontaneous generation, a hypothesis that was put forward by some as a reason for why life evolved out of chemicals. Pasteurization is the procedure that commercial food companies use the most often to eliminate bacteria from drinks and food items. However, not all colonies of bacteria are eliminated by this method.

Nowadays, pasteurization is employed in almost every packaged commercially available food item that contains substantial moisture or water amount. It includes almost every canned food that is sold on shelves or sauce, as well as mix that is placed packed in cans. These days, everything from nuts and vegetables as well as fruit, meals that are pre-packed such as meals, entrees, or chilled juices are often processed.

Pasteurization involves the processing of an ingredient to that a significant portion of bacteria is completely eliminated. There are five kinds of pasteurization: Holder steam pasteurization or steam, high temperatures or flash pasteurization ultra-high pasteurization, irradiation pasteurization, as well as gas pasteurization.

Vat, holder tunnel, steam pasteurization is the process of bringing the liquid or food item to 140-145°F over approximately 30 minutes. The majority of foods occurs in the process of heating the product following packaging. For example, cans will be heated within an airtight, sealed container. It could be followed by additional kettle cooking, and "hot-filling."

Pasteurization using steam or tunnels is used to make many drinks and sauces, particularly the ones that are packaged in glass. At this point, the food item could be heating and then hot packed. After filling the jar, the or container is then sealed. It's then placed onto a conveyor belt that is then pushed through a tunnel that is heated. The tunnel is used to bake the product and hot water sprays on the packaging. The result is a layer of steam hot inside the tunnel. This heats up the contents of the packaging and package until the right temperature. After the steam is hot, the cooling portion of the tunnel sprays colder, more refreshing water over it to help allow the product to cool down.

Flash, also known as high pasteurization (also known as HTST, which means "high temperature, short time") is carried out mostly on slurry or liquid products. HTST can bring the liquid from 160 to 165° for fifteen minutes. In some liquids, the temperature and duration is dependent on the liquid. Normal milk (non-UHT) such as is usually pasteurized through the heating process to 120°C within 20 minutes. The process is usually accomplished through pipes as well as heat exchanger plates which increase the temperature of the product quickly.

After that it is then filled with the contents of the container. A few processors still run the product through a second heating tunnel following packing to ensure that there is no contamination inside the container. Be aware that the phrase "flash pasteurized" has been employed in advertising to suggest that the system is less harmful as high temperature pasteurization.

Ultra Pasteurization (UP) can heat the liquid to up to 200° F within a couple of minutes. The time and temperature may vary according to the type of product and the final result you want. Ultra pasteurization can double shelf life of the product compared with regular pasteurization.

Also, there's ultra-high temperature pasteurization which is also known as UHT. UHT typically heats the liquid or food item at around 280° F and last for the duration of a quarter-second up to about two or three minutes. It is typically used in the case of liquids. They go through a variety of chambers that exchange extreme heat prior to being packed within an aseptic packaging. UHT is typically used to allow products to stay in a dry storage area for a longer period. It is sometimes mistakenly called sterilization.

The use of irradiation is becoming a popular technique for removing microorganisms from foods and other goods. Since it doesn't raise temperatures of the products in the same way as other techniques It is sometimes advertised by the name of "cold pasteurization."

Irradiation is another method of killing microorganisms--often employed as shipments arrive by air or by sea.

In increasing numbers, major U.S. food producers irradiate their products in order to preserve the flavor and appearance of the food is usually more appealing when it's preserved. The most popular method is cobalt-60 radiation. Gamma and X-rays are also utilized. Radiation isn't permitted for organic products. Health of workers in radiation plants is also a major concern.

Gas pasteurization is a method used in some food items. Almonds as well as other nuts as an example, are often processed by gazing them using propane oxide, or steam that is hot. Organic production of nuts is, naturally, one that doesn't allow propylene oxide.

for milk and different liquids UHT as well as HTST include homogenization. Homogenization mixes and blends with the liquid in a significant way, and could alter the molecular polarity as well as the structure.

Commercially produced foods with higher acidity (usually having a pH lower than 4.6) or a high sugar content might be allowed to avoid pasteurization. Commercial producers typically have to pass a testing for pH before they are able to pack a liquid without the need for pasteurization.

The majority of acidic juices such as orange carrot, apple, or berries were once readily available in the market as freshly. In the 1990s, following an apple juice crisis, many regulators started requiring HTST to be refrigerated fresh fruit juices.

Raw milk was readily accessible commercially for a number of years prior to the recent years. In the past, before government regulators been increasingly limiting or banning the commercial sale of packaged raw products, milk from the raw was an extremely natural probiotic drink.

Some of the last products that are not pasteurized include balsamic vinegar, tea kombucha honey, hummus and maple syrup, as well as many other probiotic-fermented items.

It is possible to ask how the probiotic and fermented foods be able to stay out of pasteurization? because they've been acidified naturally by probiotic bacteria in a way which hinders the proliferation of foodborne microbes. We'll discuss this later. probiotics eat carbohydrates and sugars and release healthy acids. They also keep pathogenic organisms away.

Chapter 16: Is Pasteurized Food Healthy?

Though this might be away from the norm however, it's a crucial issue. The majority of nutrients are sensitive to heat. Vitamin C as well as fat-soluble vitamins B, E and B vitamins as well as certain amino acids are depleted by the process of pasteurization. The other important nutrients in plants are also depleted during the process, as are various enzymes. Proteins denature or break into smaller pieces when heated long. This can help in the absorption of amino acids, it is also a way to create unnoticed mixtures of peptides. For instance, in milk the protein whey, which is nutritious, also known as lactabumin, can denature into a variety of peptides, certain of which cannot be quickly taken in.

A study in 2008 of strawberries of the University of Applied Sciences in Switzerland found the reduction of 37% in vitamin C as well as the loss of antioxidant capacity in the process of pasteurization. An investigation conducted in 1998 by Brazil's Universidade Estadual de Maringa determined that Barbados cherries lost around 14 percent of their vitamin C amount following pasteurization. After heat treatment the vitamin C can change into dehydroascorbic acid along with the loss of bioflavonoids.

An investigation conducted in 2008 at the Spanish Cardenal Herrera University determined that glutathione peroxidase, an important antioxidant found in milk was dramatically reduced due to pasteurization. In 2006, the university also announced a study proving the lysine level was dramatically diminished by pasteurization.

A study conducted by the Universidade Federal do Rio Grande discovered that pasteurizing milk reduced Vitamin A (retinol) levels by an average of 55 micrograms, to an average 36.6 micrograms.

A research conducted by North Carolina State University in 2003 found that pasteurization of HTST drastically reduced conjugated Linoleic Acid (CLA) level, which is a key dairy product that is known to decrease cancer risk and promote healthy fat metabolism.

A study conducted in 2006 on the bayberry in the Southern Yangtze University determined that the antioxidant properties of plants such as polyphenolics and anthocyanins decreased between 12-32% after UHT pasteurization. Polyphenols are the main nutrients present in both vegetables and fruits, which confer antioxidant and anticarcinogenic benefits.

Perhaps the biggest lost from pasteurization is the the amount of enzyme in food. Plant and diary foods are a rich source of many enzymes which help in the digestion of or catalyzing nutrients and antioxidants. They include lysozymes, xanthenes as well as lipases, oxidases lactoferrins, amylases and other. Food enzymes can also stop the growth of microbes and also help to prevent products from becoming spoiled. Food enzymes are utilized by the body in a variety of ways. There are some enzymes that, for instance bromelain from papaya, and papain from pineapples, break down plaque in the arteries and decrease inflammation. The body creates several natural enzymes it also absorbs certain foodstuff enzymes, or utilizes the components of these enzymes to create fresh ones.

Pasteurization leaves drink or food with a caramelized taste as a result of the exchange of a variety of flavonoids and sugars with other compounds. For example, in milk there is an extensive change from lactose into lactulose following UHT pasteurization. Lactulose may cause cramping in the intestines nausea, vomiting and cramps.

In the case of irradiation There isn't much study on the effect it has on nutritional content, aside from some microwave-based research studies (that revealed a decrease in the amount of nutrients as well as the creation of unwanted metabolic products) However, there are some indications that radiation can alter the structure of nutrients and proteins.

Natural whole foods packaged in natural packages differ significantly than processed pasteurized foods. Whole foods that are fresh and made by plants are rich in antioxidants as well as enzymes that inhibit the capability of microorganisms develop.

The Creator also offered whole foods that have shells and peels to protect the nutrients of the food and keep microorganisms away. The outside shell and peel a little However, the density, pH and dryness--along along with the acidity in the inside of the fruit, act as a shield against most microorganisms. Because of this, the majority fruit and nuts are quickly stored for several days or weeks without posing a significant microbiological risks.

After the shell or peel has been removed, the fruit either juice or nut needs to be consumed quickly in order to avoid contamination based on the sugar content of the fruit.

Whole foods are also rich in polysaccharides as well as oligosaccharides, which combine sugars and nutrients in large molecules. They are extremely difficult for pathogenic bacteria reduce them for consumption.

After processing However, sugars break down to a smaller pieces, which allows to grow microbial colonies. Why? Simple sugars are easy energy and food sources to fungi and bacteria that are growing colonies. The processed food is vulnerable to the mass colonization of microorganisms.

In the case of milk and other milk products, the raw milk may include a variety of probiotics the mother cows produce to help keep her dairy healthy and well-balanced. As they help balance our body's microbiotics and balance our microbiome, probiotics found are found in milk can stop the growth of microorganisms and infections.

However, raw milk must be bought with care. Raw milk must be obtained from certified organic dairy that have tested on pathogenic microbes. It should also predominantly grass-fed, not grain-fed. A grass-fed organic cow is much less susceptible to many illnesses since eating grass fresh helps fight off illness, just as fresh, natural foods can help fight illness for humans.

Germ or Field?

This is the essence of the illness debate that took place over the past century as well as the center of the debate on probiotics.

A different theory was developed in the late 1860s due to Louis Pasteur's belief in the germ theory, a belief that all diseases were due to microorganisms. In order to prove his claim, Pasteur infected various animals by bacterial infections and analyzed the consequences of their death against healthy animals. He proved bacteria contribute to the pathology of certain ailments which can lead to infection far over the immune system's capability to combat.

He missed an essential element that is missing from the calculation. Our entire world is filled by infectious microorganisms that are far beyond calculations. The human body has millions of bacteria. Therefore, if both the outside and within worlds are brimming by bacteria, then why aren't the majority of us infected and constantly infected?

What is the best way to remain healthy when there are so many microbes in the world? What is the way humans could endured this giant influx of microbes over hundreds of thousands of years?

The microbiologists Antoine Bechamp and Claude Bernard who were close to Pasteur who criticized the germ theory of Pasteur. They argued that the primary reason for illness isn't the virus, but rather the surrounding environment of the body. People who develop illness, Bechamp and Bernard proposed as being those who have weak and weak immune systems.

Also A healthy, well-nourished body with an immune system that is strong and good probiotic populations is better at battling the bacteria that cause infection.

The field theory in a very simple way. Foodborne illness can cause deaths and sickness of just few individuals, but hundreds, if not thousands may actually eaten the products that are contaminated.

Actually, a lot of our food items include E. coli, Salmonella as well as a variety of other species of bacteria that do not cause people sick.

The germ theory that Pasteur proposed was able to prevail, which allowed the release of antibiotics, as well as other remedies for antiseptics throughout the course of the past century. Although many of these medications have assisted millions in overcoming ailments (after the immune system has recovered) The over-use of antibiotics has destroyed internal probiotic communities and spawned several superbugs stronger than previous types of bacteria. This means that the germ theory cure is causing more dangerous bacteria!

The Probiotic Discovery

The rapid pace of industrialization and progress towards the development of chemical medicine ignored discoveries which proved the field theory, and also proved the germ theory untrue.

The first decade of the 20th century, Ilya Ilyich Mechnikov, a Nobel Prize-winning microbiologist was able to link the long-lived nature of Bulgarian and Balkan people, along with other groups due to the consumption of fermented cows' milk or buffalos, and even reindeers. Following years of studies and study, he concluded that there were tiny microorganisms in the fermented milks that might be stimulating the immune system.

The Dr. Mechnikov worked with these microorganisms for a long time, and was also a collaborator alongside Louis Pasteur. His work in the immune system have led to the understanding the role of white blood cells as well as their capacity to Phagotize (break in pieces) the invaders.

In the end, it was his range of findings to show that infectious microorganisms can be controlled and controlled through probiotics, which work as a team in conjunction with our immune systems. In the last century, since the discoveries, many scientists follow in the footsteps of Mechnikov in search of new species and strains of probiotics, which reside not just in humans however, they also live in various animals and in different environments. The field theory has been proven beyond any doubt.

That is to say, those having healthy immune systems as well as probiotic populations are less likely to become sick due to having a tiny quantity of food items that are contaminated. The body is already stocked with E. coli and Salmonella. E. Coli is usually found in healthy colon. How come we don't get sick because of these bacteria?

This is due to the fact that our probiotic bacteria keep E. bacteria populations from getting too large. Probiotics create their own range of antimicrobial substances that can inhibit or reduce the populations of pathogenic microorganisms. This table summarizes the results of two laboratory research studies, as well as an overview of studies (Chaitow and Trenev 1990) studying the inhibition zones (or the killing distance) three probiotic strains exert an effect on pathogenic bacteria that they have selected:

Bacteria Inhibition by Selected Probiotics

Pathogen

L. acidophilus1

L. bulgaricus2

B. bifidum3

Escherichia coli

44mm

40mm

20mm

Clostridium botulinum

37mm

38mm

Not tested

Clostridium perfringens

31mm

33mm

Untested

Proteus mirabilis

39mm

45mm

Not tested

Salmonella enteridis

42mm

39mm

Not tested

Salmonella typhimurium

44mm

39mm

Untested

Salmonella typhosa

Untested

Not tested

12mm

Shigella dysenteriae

30mm

Untested

11mm

Shigella paradysenteriae

30mm

Not tested

Untested

Staphylococcus aureus

35mm

38mm

23mm

Staphylococcus Faecalis

31mm

39mm

Untested

Bacillus cereus

Not tested

Not tested

22mm

Pseudomonas fluorescens

Not tested

Untested

18mm

Mocrococcus flavis

Untested

Untested

25mm

1. Lab tests of Lactobacillus acidophilus secretion acidophilin DDS1 taken from Fernandes and co. 1988.

2. Laboratory tests on Lactobacillus bulgarricus DDS14 secretion bulgarican are adapted from Fernandes and colleagues. 1988.

3. Lab tests on Bifidobacterium bifidum 1452, adapted from Anand and colleagues. 1984.

As with animals living in forests bacteria colonies are able to limit each other's numbers. When we are healthy and in a the natural environment the body is able to store adequate probiotics and their unique antibiotic strategies that keep the majority of microorganisms out of overgrowth.

Friendly Flora Nutrition

Probiotics with healthy bacteria also aid in the treatment of their "host"--us--by in addition to warding off pathogens they also aid in nourishing us. It's a reality.

Probiotics can also be described as 'friendly since they aid us absorb food, and also produce positive nutritional supplements. Incredibly, probiotics are excellent source of vital nutritional elements.

Probiotics produce biotin, thiamin (B1) as well as the riboflavin (B2) and niacin (B3) Pantothenic acid (B5) and the pyridoxine (B6) as well as cobalamine (B12) and Vitamin A, folic acid and Vitamin K. They secrete lactic acid. aid in the digestion of minerals which require acid to absorb like magnesium, iron, copper manganese, and many more.

Indeed, the majority of the multivitamins that you can buy are made by probiotic yeast and bacteria (yes they do have probiotic yeasts which we'll talk about more in the future.)

Probiotics are essential to digestion and absorption of nutrients. They remove amino acids that are part of complex proteins as well as mid-chain fatty acids that are derived from complex fats. They assist in the breakdown of the bile acids. They aid in the conversion of polyphenols found in plant material into similar biomolecules. They aid in the process of soluble fibers being fermented which results in digestible sugars and fatty acids. Apart from other tasks that are nutritive and functions, they can also aid in enhancing calcium bioavailability.

The table below reviews beneficial effects of probiotics on nutrition within the human body.

Probiotic Nutrition

Biotin

Probiotics are the probiotics that produce it.

Thiamin (B1)

The probiotics in the diet are responsible for its production.

Riboflavin (B2)

The probiotics in the diet are responsible for its production.

Niacin (B3)

The probiotics in the diet are responsible for its production.

Pantothenic Acid (B5)

Probiotics are the probiotics that produce it.

Pyridoxine (B6)

The probiotics in the diet are responsible for its production.

Cobalamine (B12)

Probiotics are the probiotics that produce it.

Folic Acid (B9)

Probiotics are the probiotics that produce it.

Vitamin A

Probiotics are the probiotics that produce it.

Vitamin K

The probiotics in the diet are responsible for its production.

Copper

Bioavailability increases with probiotics.

Calcium

Probiotics boost bioavailability

Magnesium

Bioavailability increases with probiotics.

Iron

Bioavailability increases with probiotics.

Manganese

Probiotics boost bioavailability

Potassium

Bioavailability increases with probiotics.

Zinc

Probiotics boost bioavailability

Proteins

Probiotics break down for digestibility

Fats

Probiotics break down for digestibility

Carbohydrates

Probiotics are able to break down and help process

Sugars

Probiotics are able to break down and help process

Milk

Probiotics can improve digestibility

Phytonutrients

Probiotics improve digestion

Cholesterol

Probiotics can bind to and lower blood sugar levels

Note there are a few probiotics that do not create the same amount of nutrients. In fact, some are able to consume certain nutrients other probiotics produce. Like, for instance, Lactobacillus bulgaricus can produce folic acids in yogurt. In addition, lactobacillus acidolpholus consumes folate. When you're done with the day, any mixture of probiotics may still provide an increase in the amount of nutrition, but. This is why the majority of probiotics that are cultured have greater amounts of nutrients than cream or milk the products were created with.

They also help with peristalsis, which is the regular digestion process by aiding the flow of digestive contents through the digestive tract. Probiotics also make antifungal compounds including acidophillin and bifidin and hydrogen peroxide. These combat the growth of non-friendly yeasts. Hydroperoxide from probiotics is in turn oxygenating, facilitating antioxidants and scavenging of free radicals. Additionally, they produce vital fatty acids. They provide 5-10 percent of the short chained fats that are essential to a healthy immunity.

Probiotics indirectly and directly remove toxins by utilizing the biochemical process and colonizing. Probiotics' nutrient production has been proven to possess beneficial anticancer and antitumor effects in the body. Probiotics that are beneficial can block the absorption of harmful toxins such as mercury as well as the other metals that are heavy. Some will directly bind to the toxins, or facilitate the binding of different molecules to get rid of the toxins.

Probiotics are essential in reducing the rate of cell degeneration as well as related diseases. Because of their nutrition-related mechanisms they help to regulate the blood levels of cholesterol as well as triglycerides. Certain probiotics can even aid in breaking down and build hormones.

The probiotics can increase the effectiveness of the thymus and spleen, two most important organs in the immune system.

Probiotics are essential for proper digestion. The probiotics' populations are located in the mucosal lining creating a layer to aid in the process of filtering out and processing toxins and other material before they reach in the wall of our intestinal cells. This helps keep the brushes barrier cells, and protects the mucosal linings of our intestines free of damage due to foreign substances that come from our food items and their secondary metabolites. The damage to the cells of the brush of the intestinal lining can be the main reason behind several intestinal disorders, including irritable bowel.

In a study that demonstrates the probiotic-produced production of a essential nutrient Italian researchers offered 23 healthy participants Bifidobacterium Adolescentis, as well as Bifidobacterium pseudocatenulatum. The stool samples collected prior to and after the there was a marked increase in bioavailability of folic acids in each of the strains of probiotic.

Probiotics can also be a threat to pathogens for food sources. If they are in good quantities the strategy could reduce any potential for infection. The probiotics' nutrients aid in stimulating our immune cells in our body as well as normalize the activity of immune cells during inflammation situations.

We'll now explore this intriguing aspect of probiotics - their connection to our body's immune system.

Chapter 17: The Probiotic Immune System

Probiotics in our body make up around 70 percentage of our immune response. The title of this chapter proves the crucial role that probiotics play in our immune system. However, the actual picture inside is more amazing. We will learn more about this in the subsequent chapters, probiotic colonies interact in conjunction with the immune system in your body to increase the number of immune cells and antibodies which identify and destroy infective microorganisms.

Before diving into the details of the role played by probiotics in the fight against infection, we'll take an overview of our immune system:

When a person removes a human heart from a dead body, and transferred into a live human body, its immune system instantly begins to block the heart. The reason for this is that the body's immune system is aware of the heart as not being an integral part within the human body. What does it mean?

The immune system exists all over the body. The immune system is found on our skin, within the bloodstream, in the lungs, inside the bones, as well as in each organ system. Additionally, we find the immune system inside millions of probiotics spread throughout the body.

The immune system is equipped with several intelligent capacities. One of them is the recognition. The immune system is equipped with the capability to identify compounds that can harm the wellbeing of the body. The immune system is also able to keep memories.

The immune system has the ability to recognize the specificity of a toxins or pathogen through being able to recognize the antibodies (byproducts or molecular components). This is why we recommend vaccination. The body is exposed to the smallest amount specific pathogens, and the immune system can develop the necessary tools and memories to recognize the antigens it has, in order to react appropriately next time it comes in contact to the pathogen.

It is amazing with its capacity to preserve the specificity and variety. This allows the immune system to millions, perhaps billions, of antigens. Furthermore, every antigen has a distinct reaction.

The immune system functions as an intelligent scan review and re-reading system designed to identify whether a certain body, molecule or even organism can be found in our body. It does this by using an intricate biochemical identification process.

This system could be compared with fingerprint recognition. With the database of fingerprints an individual is recognized with their fingerprints, in the event that their fingerprints appear in the system.

The same is true for the immune system examines molecular structure against its own database. If the molecular structure can't be recognised, or does not match the structure that's considered to be foreign the immune system initiates an attack. The attack is known as an immune response, or an inflammation reaction.

While there is a lot of research being conducted on vaccines, antibiotics and inflammation, the modern medical field is still a bit baffled by auto-immune condition. An array of diseases that are classed as autoimmune. This includes Crohn's disease, irritable bowel syndrome as well as allergies, asthma and fibromyalgia. They also have lupus or urinary tract problems as well as many more. Doctors classify the majority of forms that are arthritis as auto-immune diseases.

How can the immune system be able to heal these conditions, just as it has done with many other kinds of injuries? What's wrong within our immune system?

In terms of infections bacteria, harmful microbes and chemicals infiltrate the body through the digestive tract, nasal and sinuses, genitals and the lungs, external skin, the ears as well as the eyes. Infections caused by bacteria can occur due to normal resident within the human body.

A healthy body is healthier in the event that toxins or harmful bacteria outnumber their healthy levels, the immune system -- which includes of probiotics -- will launch an attack on our colon.

www.ingramcontent.com/pod-product-compliance
Lightning Source LLC
Chambersburg PA
CBHW060222030426
42335CB00014B/1314